The Best of
The Rogue Nutritionist

V O L U M E   I

Jonny Bowden, PhD., CNS

TABLE OF CONTENTS

DIET SECRETS OF THE HOLLYWOOD STARS 7

DEBUNKING THE MYTH OF THE FAT BURNING ZONE 11

DO WE REALLY NEED VITAMIN SUPPLEMENTS? 15

WHY DID I EAT THAT CHEESECAKE? 19

LOSING MOTIVATION 23

6 GREAT MOTIVATIONAL TIPS 28

8 WAYS TO BREAK A PLATEAU 36

THE ASPARTAME CONTROVERSY 40

AFFORDABLE NUTRITION 44

5 BEST FOODS TO FUEL YOUR WORKOUT 48

CRITIQUING YOUR INNER CRITIC 52

AIRPORT EATING 57

FOOD OVERDOSE.. 61

7 TIPS FOR HOLIDAY EATING 65

FOOD AND LOVE.. 69

7 IMPOSTERS: HEALTHY FOODS THAT AREN'T........... 72

THE ETERNAL TRUTHS OF DIETING 75

FOOD DIARIES AND JOURNALS..................................... 81

IS YOUR INNER CRITIC HOLDING YOU BACK? 85

EAT YOUR WAY TO WELLNESS IN SIX EASY STEPS...... 89

10 SUPERFOODS YOU NEED TO KNOW ABOUT 93

IT'S ALL ABOUT THE CALORIES, RIGHT? 97

WHY STRESS MATTERS 101

FALLING OFF THE DIET WAGON................................ 105

DIET SECRETS OF THE HOLLYWOOD STARS

Oh, did I ever know that headline would get your attention.

OK, are you really, *really* ready for the real, true, honest dirt? The complete truth about Hollywood diet secrets? I promise you, this is the *real deal*, and I'm going to back it up with hard evidence, so get set to take notes. Here's the real, serious-business truth about the dieting secrets of the Hollywood stars:

There are none.

Want proof? I compiled the following from recent interviews and articles on the dieting "secrets" of Hollywood stars: Alicia Silverstone is a vegan. Joan Lunden eats fruit. Jennifer Anniston is on the Zone. Dianne Sawyer does cabbage soup. Heather Locklear likes McDonalds and french fries. Jennifer Lopez eats eight mini-meals. Claudia Schiffer sips green tea. Patricia Heaton eats lots of dairy. Melanie Griffith drinks smoothies. Demi Moore eats high-protein. Nia Peebles shuns protein. Kelly Preston eats oatmeal and bagels.

In other words, as the brilliant writer William Goldman once said about Hollywood....

"Nobody knows anything".

In fact, the only remotely sensible statement I found anywhere in researching this column was one by Sarah Michelle Geller who basically said "look, it's crazy for people to try to be as thin as we are. We have personal trainers and personal chefs. It's our *job* to look this way"

Even then, folks, it ain't easy. Check out some of those "candid" photos of the stars when they're not made up and done up and dressed up and are just relaxing on the beach not realizing they're being stalked by some paparazzi with a 500mm telephoto lens and a contract with the tabloids.

No, we'd love to believe that everyone in Hollywood has the magic secret and if only we could figure out what it was, we too could look like they do. Nice theory, but it has a few holes in it.

Number one: There's no "they". Hollywood stars come in all shapes and sizes and metabolic and genetic types just like we do, they have varying degrees of addiction just like we do, they have varying degrees of discipline and motivation just like we do, and they respond completely differently to different regimens. Just like we do.

Number two: They don't know any more than we do. Most go to their friends or hairdressers for diet tips, or get introduced to the latest diet guru because they share the same publicist. Some stars hire people to tell them what to do, and the people they hire are as different in their approaches and as varied in their skills as any group of experts on diet and nutrition anywhere. Which is to say a lot. Sure some trainers or nutritionists become "hot" for a while, just like a hairstylist does, but they get "not hot" faster than the wardrobe changes at the Radio City Christmas Show. I've seen a dozen come into favor and go out faster than you can say "the E True Hollywood Story".

Number three: They struggle with the same issues about food and drink, and their bodies respond in the same variety of ways. The only differences are that they do it in full view of the public and that they have access to magicians- called hair, make-up and lighting people- to do things to them that you simply can't believe unless you've seen it done in front of your very eyes. I have, and I can tell you this: what these folks can do makes the Siegfried and Roy Show look like a card trick.

Once in a while, a star will lend her name to a diet book, or a workout video. Most often, if it's any good, it was designed by someone else. The star may have some input, just like they do when they do a signature line perfume, but you didn't really think Elizabeth Taylor sat there and blended 65 notes of fragrance, did you? Cindy Crawford's first video was designed by NY trainer Radu. Cher's was done by Keli Roberts. And the popular Sommersizing books are basically modified versions of the Schwarzbein Principle by Dr. Diana Schwarzbein who was her advisor on the project. (But Suzanne *does* look great on the book jacket.)

Now this is not a put-down to Hollywood stars. I've known many of them and they're very nice people. Or at least some are. But they are not the best people to turn to for nutritional advice. Look, it's hard enough to find a nutritionist who knows what he or she is doing. Why would you expect biochemistry expertise from Gwyneth Paltrow?

There *is* one secret to Hollywood diets, and it's the same secret I've been telling my Diet Boot Campers for years now. It's the only secret you'll ever need to know, and if you really get it and accept it, you'll be on the way to success not only in weight loss but in life. Here it is:

Everybody's different.

Oh by the way, 'case you were interested. Mel Gibson doesn't eat chicken.

Wanna know why?

He read somewhere that men who eat chicken breasts run the risk of sprouting breasts themselves.

Questions, anyone?

DEBUNKING THE MYTH OF THE FAT BURNING ZONE

Are you ready for the top ten things to know about the "fat burning zone", that mysterious place determined by obscure heart rate formulas that tell you exactly where you should be exercising in order to "burn" the most fat?

OK, here's number one: It's a lie.

If you're still curious about the other nine things to know, read on….

Like an urban legend that just won't die, the idea of the ideal "fat burning zone" continues to survive every reasonable attempt by exercise physiologists and nutritionists to explain to the general public why the concept is at best misleading. To be fair, their mission is not exactly helped by treadmill manufacturers who insist on putting "fat burning" programs on their machines, nor is it helped by the legions of aerobic teachers who neither understand the physiology nor can do the math.

So let's give the truth another try.

"Fat burning" is actually a vernacular expression, a "shorthand" for what exercise professionals refer to as "the beta oxidation of fatty acids". And therein lies part of the confusion. When we regular people talk about "fat burning" we have in our minds some vague concept of cellulite literally melting in a furnace of exercise-induced body heat. In fact, what happens is a little different.

At any given moment in time, you are "burning" (or, technically, "oxidizing") fuel (food), breaking it down for energy. The food you eat- carbohydrates, fats, proteins-gets taken apart by the body, broken down into its smallest components (fatty acids, amino acids and glucose respectively) which provide energy for the body to do anything and everything that it needs to do. That means providing energy to grow nails and hair, to breathe, to make enzymes, to digest food, to exercise, think, sit at the computer, garden, run for the bus and even sleep. The particular *mix* of fuel that it uses depends on a number of things.

And therein lies the rub.

See, at rest, the greatest *proportion* of your fuel comes from fat. So in theory, if you wanted to "burn" the most fat, you would simply stay in bed. The "fuel split" then would be, theoretically, about 70 per cent "fat" and 30 per cent "carbohydrate" (let's leave protein out of the equation for the moment.. the body prefers to use protein for other things, and won't ordinarily use it for energy unless it has to). Why then don't you lose any weight just staying in bed?

Because, even though the lion's share of the calories burned by just staying in bed does indeed come from fat, the *total amount of calories burned* is tiny. In other words, you're burning a *high percentage* of a very small number (about 1 calorie a minute in the "average" person).

Now, what happens when you begin to exercise?

Well, the minute you start to move from a resting position, the "fuel split" changes… carbohydrate starts to contribute a slightly greater percentage of the mix, and fat a slightly smaller one. The greater the intensity of the exercise, the greater the *proportion* of calories from carbohydrate and the smaller the *proportion* of calories from fat. But.. and this is a big important but… the harder the exercise, the greater the total number of calories per minute. So although your *percentage* from fat goes down, your *total number* increases.

Every Internet baby who has ever invested in a start-up understands this concept perfectly. Each time you bring in more investors for your company, the *percentage* that you own of the company decreases, but the *value* of the company goes way up. So, for example, instead of owning 10 percent of a company worth a million, you now own only 5 percent - but of a company that's suddenly worth *six* million. Do the math and tell me- which would you rather have?

This is where your average aerobics teacher gets it all mixed up. By telling you to keep your heart rate low no matter what, they're essentially admonishing you to keep your "fat percentage" high… but without considering that *the less intense exercise also burns a smaller total number of calories.*

If you think I'm telling you to exercise harder, you're right. But with a caveat. If you're new to exercising, there are a lot of reasons to keep your heart rate in a reasonably low zone. First, you're less likely to become exhausted and quit (and what good is burning a ton of calories a minute if you can only keep it up for one minute?). Second, you're less likely to get injured. Third, all things being equal, a long bout of slow exercise will "burn" as many calories as a short bout of intense exercise, plus it will begin to train the fat mobilizing enzymes to come out of hiding.

What you don't want to lose sight of, however, is that exercising at a higher level of intensity has a lot of benefits as well. For one thing, it increases your aerobic capacity and conditions your heart. For another, it burns a ton of calories. For a third, it pushes your "threshold", making you fitter and more conditioned- and a more *conditioned* person is a more efficient "fat burner" during her non-exercising hours.

And ultimately, fuel is like money. Does it really matter if you pay your rent with five dollar bills, twenty dollar bills, or hundred dollar bills? One way or another, you're going to take some money out of your bank account, and, when you exercise, one way or another you're going to burn up some "savings". Whether they happen to come from carbohydrates or fat matters very little in the scheme of things. If you keep your carbohydrate intake moderate, and you burn an excess of calories on a regular basis, eventually guess where that excess is going to come out of?

Exactly. So throw out those fat burning charts, and use the following rule instead: Within the limits of your ability and fitness level, and without causing undue stress or increasing the possibility of injury, *exercise as hard and as long as you can, as frequently as you can.*

That and the right diet and you've got the recipe for success.

DO WE REALLY NEED VITAMIN SUPPLEMENTS?

OK, first a confession. If you came to my house and looked in my kitchen cabinets, you might well think I'm nuts. There are at least 75 bottles of different supplements, powders, green drinks, vitamins, minerals and other assorted potions. Now I confess, I don't take all of them every day. But that's because some are duplicates- in a rare display of personal organization, I keep a couple of extra vitamin C's and B's and the like because I run out so fast. But I do probably consume, oh, I don't know, somewhere in the neighborhood of (gasp) fifty supplements a day.

"What" you cry? "Are you nuts?". Go ahead and laugh. I've heard it all before. I don't mind. I realize my routine isn't for everyone. But before you write me off as certifiable, let me round out the picture for you.

Look in my medicine cabinet for prescription drugs. It's empty. No antihistamines, pain killers, blood pressure meds, cholesterol lowerers, antacids, Nexium, or any of the myriad of other pills folks "my age" consume on a regular basis. Next look through my doctor bills. If you can find them. About the only time I see doctors is when I meet my friends at the nutritional medicine conferences or when I interview them for articles. I get sick almost never, and when I do, I recover in about 1/10 the time it takes everyone else around me to recover from the same "bug".

Now do I attribute all this to vitamins? Not exactly. (More on that in future columns). But I'll tell you this: My energy, sleep habits, mood, optimism, vitality and general health has never been better, and I'm not messing with a winning formula.

Which brings us to the subject at hand: *Do you need to take vitamins?*

Glad you asked.

One of the things I'm asked about the most is supplements. First, do we need them? Second, what do they *do* anyway? Third, can any of them help with weight loss? Fourth, can't we get all the vitamins we need from a balanced diet? Fifth, how do we pick the most important ones? And sixth, what the heck do they do anyway (yes I know I mentioned that one before, but just wanted to see if you were paying attention).

Those are all great questions, and in future columns (and books) I'll discuss the answers to all of them and more. But for now, let's just now, let me just whet your appetite a bit. Let's just tackle the first one: do we need the darn things in the first place?

In the best of all possible worlds, you should theoretically be able to get "all you need" from food. There are two "operative phrases" here: first is "best of all possible worlds", second is "all you need". Let's examine both.

This is *not* the best of all possible worlds. That world- which doesn't exist- would be one in which there was no stress, no pollution (not in the soil, water supply or air), no toxins for our bodies to get rid of, and everyone ate organically grown food which we got from our own natural gardens. Further, we'd eat around the family dinner table each night with no television, bonding with our family members, after which we'd all retire as the sun went down to a nice deep sleep of at least eight hours in length. Hey while I'm dreaming, let's throw world peace into the mix. And humane treatment for all sentient beings including animals.

Needless to say, that's not reality. Reality is that our daily lives present us with dozens of challenges all of which have profound implications for our health. Stress eats up vitamins. So does lack of sleep (neurotransmitters and hormones aren't rebuilt and replaced). Special conditions- age, pregnancy, athletics- put special demands on the body. The soil our food is grown in is depleted of nutrients. The meat we eat has a ton of steroids, antibiotics and hormones. The medicines we take have to be detoxed by our overworked livers, already reeling from the toxic burden of what's in the air and water and sprayed on our food. Need I go on?

I didn't think so.

So let's move on to the second "operative phrase, "all you need".

The dietitians and nutritionally uninformed medical experts who continue to preach that we can get "all we need" in the way of vitamins and minerals from food are right- *if* you're talking about preventing nutritional deficiencies like beriberi and rickets. Don't know about you, but I've never seen a case of scurvy. Preventing diseases of nutritional deficiency- which are pretty darn rare in America- should hardly be the goal of vitamin and mineral intake. I call that "minimum wage nutrition".

I'm not interested in "minimum wage nutrition". I'm interested in optimal health and well-being. I'm interested in you being as great as you can be in the world, in health *and* in life. And to achieve that, why would you not use every tool at your disposal?

Supplements are simply a technology to deliver nutrients your body needs to perform virtually every metabolic task in it's repertoire. Why would we not avail ourselves of that technology to feed our bodies the optimal dosages of the nutrients it needs to run on? In dosages not necessarily to prevent deficiency, but to create optimal well-being?

After all, remember: Depression is not a Prozac deficiency!

WHY DID I EAT THAT CHEESECAKE?

I recently received an email asking the following question:

> "How come even old fitness veterans have such a hard time staying on the healthy eating track?"

The writer went on to detail her own personal battles with food with certain situations being particularly problematic. For her, these situations included being on vacation, eating with her family, and especially, attending social events.

Her question is profoundly familiar to virtually anyone who has ever struggled with weight. This was a person who had experienced great success with my Diet Boot Camp program and understood the principles really well, yet, like many people, she kept "falling off the wagon", and when she did, she found it difficult to get back on track. She wondered if I had any thoughts on the subject.

Sure I do. And one of them is this: *I think it's darn near a miracle that it doesn't happen more often!*

Here's why: If information was all that was needed to change our lives, all any of us would need to do is read some books and we'd be good to go. Do smokers hold on to their cigarettes away because someone forgot to tell them it causes lung cancer? If all we needed to do good things was good information, it would be pretty easy to do all sorts of stuff: walk away from bad relationships, lower our stress levels, drop a little weight, stop drinking, you name it. Clearly a lot more is going on here than just knowing the facts.

There are powerful forces that can often seem like they're conspiring to work against you when you attempt to change your eating behavior patterns. Remember the ancient wisdom of the warrior: Know thine enemy. Understanding these forces can help lessen their power over you. At the very least, understanding them can help you be a little easier on yourself if you find yourself not always sticking on the "straight and narrow".

I'm going to give you a preview of the five biggest obstacles to changing the way you eat and staying with your plan. Next, I'll explain each of them in more depth, and also tell you about one particular *good* "reason" to occasionally give yourself a treat.

The five biggest obstacles:
1) Habits and Conditioning
2) Food Allergies / Hypersensitivities
3) Brain Chemistry
4) Genetic Factors
5) The Food Supply Itself

Habits and Conditioning. Eating behavior begins to be conditioned the moment we're out of the womb. Food is strongly associated with all kinds of social situations, rituals, places, people and emotions- not the least of which is comfort. These responses are powerfully conditioned over a lifetime-- they don't just "go away" in a few weeks or even months. You might as well expect that there are going to be times when a particular constellation of those factors- people, places, things and emotions- will simply overwhelm even the best "intentions".

Food Allergies/Hypersensitivities. This is the "betcha can't eat just one syndrome". Foods to which we are reactive or hypersensitive produce a response in the body which is followed by the release of endorphins, the body's own natural painkillers. These endorphins make you feel good. It's very very easy to become "addicted" to foods like this. They're like cigarettes to a smoker. Those cigarettes aren't good for the body, and the first time you smoke one you will choke. But once you adapt to the "damage", you're hooked. And if you quit and then pick up again, what happens? You want them all the time. And the foods that cause the most problems are usually the same foods that are most "tempting" during outings, vacations, and other

Brain Chemistry. Our desires for food are strongly influenced by neurotransmitters like serotonin. When serotonin levels are depressed or depleted, we're very subject to cravings (think: PMS!) Stress plays a part too, as high levels of cortisol (a stress hormone) can cause us to crave carbohydrates

Genetic Factors. Although we're far from having a complete understanding of this one, there is virtually no one on the planet who doesn't believe that lurking in the genome are at least some genes that have an effect on appetite and weight gain. There is undoubtedly a genetic component that makes it easier for certain people to put weight on and harder for those same people to lose it. There may be a genetically determined "range" of weight that your body "likes" to stay in. And while some people can indeed get out of that range, don't expect to do it without a bit of resistance from the universe!

A completely out-of-control toxic food supply. On a yearly basis, you are exposed to somewhere in the neighborhood of 90,000 advertisements for food, most of it horrible. And that doesn't count the daily, crushing, unrelenting exposure to restaurants, malls, food courts, magazine photos, radio spots, billboards, snack machines, buffets, office luncheons, pizza huts, Chinese take-out, overflowing supermarket aisles, Starbucks and Dunkin Donuts. The food industry spends hundreds of millions of dollars attempting to make the culinary equivalent of a toxic waste dump seem appealing, refreshing, healthy, fresh and delicious to you, so much so that it has actually convinced you that to not eat this junk is "deprivation".

So, are there "reasons" why people "fall off the wagon"? You bet there are. But rather than beat yourself up for occasionally "giving in", or for losing "only a couple" of pounds, I would prefer to see you congratulate yourself for what you *have* done, and *are doing*!

In this environment, the fact that you are able to resist junk at all, lose any weight and regain any measure of health is a tribute to your strength and your ability to be empowered.

By the way there's one other reason, and, when it's not "contaminated" by excess baggage from the other five, it's a perfectly fine reason to "stray", and not one I'm sure I want to give up: It's called pleasure. Simply put, there *is* a place for recreational eating and for sampling delicious, sinful treats from time to time. As long as you can make it work for you, as long as it's not compulsive or destructive, as long as it's not being fueled by boredom, sadness, anger, or any of the other pyramid of reasons people eat badly, and as long as it serves *you* rather than you serving *it*, I say go for it. I know of no better reason to have a treat.

LOSING MOTIVATION

"About five years ago I was in the best shape of my life -- then I got involved in an abusive relationship and ended up gaining 40 pounds ... I would like to start working out again, but every time I try, I lose motivation, give up and become more depressed."

Do you have your own version of this question, which I get asked- in some form or another- on a regular basis?

If so, read on.

I once had the pleasure of knowing Rob Kapilow, one of the great young conductors in America who also happens to be an enormously gifted teacher. One day he told me that he had just been called by the Boston Opera Company to come in and be a last minute replacement for an ailing conductor. He needed to conduct a Verdi opera, (they're *very* long), which he was not familiar with. Not only that, it was in a language which he did not speak. Not only that, the conducting gig was in four days. He basically had a weekend to learn the piece.

By the way, the Boston Opera does not suffer fools gladly,

if you get my drift.

Rob was completely sanguine.

When I heard this story, I was incredulous. How are you going to learn this piece in time? I asked. Already I was reeling from the sheer enormity of the task, the impossibility of it and the anxiety that would have to be associated with not only learning it, but being able to lead some very craggy, cynical musicians in its performance. And it was not even my gig.

Simple, he said with a shrug. I'll learn it the same way I learn any piece.

One bar at a time.

That simple four word statement taught me everything I ever needed to know about motivation and accomplishment.

See, it's not the *task*- getting in shape, losing forty pounds- that's defeating you, it's your *perception* of it. You're being defeated by allowing yourself to feel the sheer "enormity" of the full opera, so to speak. That's exactly what most of us do when confronted with changing our bodies. What's interesting to me is that we often don't do it in other arenas of our lives.

For example, if you decide to have a child, do you consider the huge task of the next eighteen years, from the number of hours it will take each day to nurse her and watch after her while she's an infant to the amount of money it will take to send her to college?

If you went to university, did you look at the whole four years and think of the number of books you'd have to read, the amount of material you need to learn, the number of tests you'd have to pass in order to get that degree?

Probably not. No, in both cases, though you might have glanced down the road at the bigger picture, you probably did the day-to-dayness of it one day at a time.

Or, in Rob's case, one bar at a time.

And if you are to be successful in your current goal, you're going to have to do it the same way.

One pound at a time.

See, our subconscious minds are very stupid, very digital. They only understand two states: on and off, yes and no, success and failure. No one on the planet likes to continue an activity in which they always fail. That's why, when we undertake weight loss or body transformation, we need to trick ourselves into winning, at least until we're hooked. It's like playing a game with a kid. You don't throw the ball too far or too hard or the kid will never catch it and will have a terrible time and give up. Instead, you "cheat" so that the kid can win. Once the kid gets good and loves the game, then you can make it harder.

Well, that's what you've got to do with yourself right now. You've got to treat your subconscious mind like that kid and "trick" it into winning.

How do you do that? Simple.

You set up goals that are preposterously, stupendously easy. Things at which you cannot possibly fail. Maybe it's walking for one minute. Maybe it's just going to the gym, and not even changing into workout clothes. Maybe it's doing three minutes on a treadmill. Maybe it's watching the first four minutes of a Tae-Bo tape from your living room couch.

Think that's silly? Think again.

Remember that your subconscious doesn't evaluate big or little, it only knows success or failure. If you tell yourself you're going to do 30 minutes of aerobics and you only do 27, that's logged as a failure. Couple of those and you "lose motivation" and are out of the game. But if you tell yourself you're going to do 3 minutes, and you actually do them, it's recorded as a success. You leave the game a winner.

Now the trick is to do that every day. Why? To build up the habit of believing your own word. The one take home point from this is that it *does not matter what you do, it matters only that you do it.* And that you do "it" successfully. That your subconscious scores it as a 'win'. So set it up so that it's impossible to fail. Don't worry about it if the goal you set seems ridiculously easy. That's OK; you'll be upping the bar soon enough. Remember that the prime goal here is not the amount of exercise you do or how "good" you are on your "diet"; the prime goal here is to develop a new habit: *doing what you say you're going to do.* Whatever that is. Fill in the blanks. You can always up the ante later. If you start with one minute and add a minute a day, in a month you'll be doing a half hour.

So bypass the "no motivation" blockade by forgetting about the enormity of the goal. Instead, all you need is enough motivation to do one minute.

The pounds will come off, your body will change, and your motivation will grow.

The same way Rob learned the Verdi opera.

One bar at a time.

6 GREAT MOTIVATIONAL TIPS

From time to time—OK, OK, everyday—I'm asked for tips about motivation. Here's what I think: Motivation comes and goes. It's just a feeling. It's lovely to have, sure, and you get all inspired and busy when you have it, but the fact is you can't count on it. Motivation is really just about "feelin' it", and truth be told, you ain't always gonna be "feelin' it". The real action is in taking a stand for yourself and making a commitment to do something whether you feel like it or not.

I didn't wait to "feel like it" to stop smoking cigarettes. If I had, I'd probably be puffing on a Marlboro as I write this. And if you're married, you probably didn't say in your vows "I promise to be with this person for as long as... I feel like it". No. You take a stand, and then you live into that stand, whether you feel like it or not. That way you don't have to depend on a fleeting feeling of inspiration that, while it's great to have, shouldn't be the only source of fuel to drive your behavior.

Remember, some writers achieve greatness not by waiting for a burst of inspiration, but by setting a definite schedule where they sit in front of the computer even if not a single word comes to their mind. The discipline and commitment to do it anyway—even if motivation is temporarily absent-is what gets the job done.

So in my view, the best "motivational tips" are those that help you set the stage for success. In "Unleash Your Thin" we call them "intention actions"—like setting out a water bottle before bed so you remember to take it with you in the morning. If you make it easier for yourself to act, you may not need to depend so much on something unreliable like "motivation".

Instead you'll come to depend on something much more powerful: Yourself.

1. <u>Bulletproof your kitchen</u>

Know what the first step in any twelve-step program is? Admitting that you're powerless over whatever it is you're addicted to. And that goes for food as well.

There's a lot of power in admitting powerlessness, because it opens up possibilities for action If there are certain situations- or in this case, foods- that you have a lot of trouble with, *get rid of them.* Bulletproof your kitchen. Why tempt fate? I personally can't eat one small portion of ice cream and put the rest away, so guess what I do? I don't keep ice cream in the house! Simple. Set yourself up for success by ridding your immediate environment of the stuff you have a hard time with. If it's not there, there's much less chance you'll eat it. And If you live with other people, ask their cooperation or make a separate area of the kitchen that's just for you—and make the rest of the stuff in the kitchen off-limits.

Bulletproofing your kitchen is the first step towards setting yourself up for success. And by the way, why stop with the kitchen? Take the lesson you learned about toxic foods and apply it to the rest of your life. Make a list of those "toxic friends", "toxic situations" and "energy drainers" in your life and start cleaning house. You have enormous personal power to create an environment that supports you in your goals, whether it be weight loss or stress reduction or anything else you want for yourself.

Start using it now. Start with the kitchen- but don't stop there!

2. Watch your language!

You ever notice that when you say "I'm having a really bad day" things just seem to get worse?

Our language is very powerful and actually influences our reality. The way we *frame* things- the language we use to describe experience- is a very important tool that most of us don't take advantage of. Saying "I'm fat", or "I have no willpower", or "I'll never be thin" are all statements that *close off* possibilities rather than open them. Those statements send a message to your powerful unconscious that "this is the way things are".

Bad move. Studies have shown that our thoughts have powerful influences on our outcomes. Start framing your reality in *positive* terms- visualize yourself at the weight you want to be and *write it down.*

Use affirmation statements- like "I am 135 pounds and enjoying wonderful, vibrant health!" and put those statements on 3x5 cards and post them where you can see them every day. Even if they're not real for you yet, those positive images and thoughts send powerful messages to your subconscious that may influence the choices you make going forward.

3. Write down your goals

Consider this: Two people want to go on vacation. One says to the travel agent, "just get me on a plane somewhere out of here". The other says, "I want to go to St. Martin in December, I want to stay on the French side of the island, and I want daily time booked with the tennis pro".

Who do you think is more likely to have a great vacation?

Now ask yourself why.

The second person wins because he's very specific about what he wants. That's the first step towards getting it, but most of us don't do it. So here's a tip we can learn from winners-- be very *specific* about what you want, and then *write it down*! Virtually every successful person has some system for doing this. You should too.

And when you write those goals down, do it in a very specific, positive way. Don't just say "I want to lose some weight" or "I'd like to be thin". Pick a specific goal weight, a specific date and a specific time, and then frame it in a positive way. For example, "I weigh 140 pounds at 5 PM on May 31st". Actually *see* and *feel* yourself experiencing that. You can do that with goals in every area of your life.

The more specific you are and the more positively you frame it, the greater likelihood of you actually seeing it happen.

4. Acknowledge someone

Here's a tip that will not only change your life, but will make a difference to the people around you: Acknowledge someone. Every single day. Here's why:

Most people in the world just want to make a difference. They want to contribute. And they want to be acknowledged for the contributions they make. Think about it: don't you? How do you feel when someone tells you you're doing a great job?

I thought so.

But here's the thing: Acknowledging doesn't just make a difference for the person being acknowledged. It makes a difference for the person *doing* the acknowledging as well. Which in this case is you. Don't you feel better when you're delivering good news? Every time you tell someone what they mean to you, it not only brightens their day, it brightens yours. And acknowledging- a close cousin to gratitude- helps you focus on the things that are good and wonderful in your life.

The acknowledgement can be small- like telling the elevator operator what great taste in hats he has- or it can be huge. Point is to do it. You can even spend a minute or two thanking your animal companions for the adorable and lovable things they do or for the joy they bring into your life. Doesn't matter: just express it. In some small way, acknowledging changes your life. It's a great habit to cultivate. Do it every day this holiday season and watch what happens.

5. <u>Make friends with your juicer</u>

I frequently give a talk to groups called "Nutritional Immunity" where I talk about all the things we can do to strengthen our immune system, a popular topic these days. Of course, immunity being what it is, and me being who I am, I eventually get around to the role stress and anxiety has in immunity, and the interpersonal and lifestyle choices we can make to create a better life, which in turn decreases the stress hormone cortisol, which in turn increases immunity- well, you get the idea.

And at the end of the talk, I leave them with one tip: Make friends with your juicer. And if you don't have a juicer, buy one. Here's why:

Live, raw food- like fruits and vegetables- is loaded with enzymes. It also contains some of the most potent cocktails of antioxidants, phytochemicals, flavanoids, and other unpronounceable health-giving, DNA-protecting nutrients you can possibly imagine. That's why we nutritionists are constantly telling everyone to eat their vegetables and fruits. But let's be honest- a lot of people aren't doing it. Certainly not in the quantities we recommend. But I've yet to see even the most vegetable-phobic person (including teenagers) turn down a glass of freshly made juice.

Fresh juice is naturally sweet- especially when you use apples and/or carrots as a base- and you can throw in such teenage kryptonite as broccoli and they won't even notice. Nor will you. The juice is filling, delicious, and you can experiment with a zillion combinations including (but not limited to) beets, spinach, celery, parsley, ginger and just about anything in the produce section.

And for some unknown reason, after a filling glass of freshly made juice, the chocolate ice cream or cake seems less appealing.

Juice from a juicer is a natural healthy weight loss food that knocks the socks off any weight loss supplement on the market, and gives you cancer-fighting, life-giving nutrients as well. I start every single day with a freshly made juice. Try it- it's health in a glass.

6. Ask four questions*

When I do weight loss programs, I rarely concentrate on diet and exercise alone. To me, weight loss is like a stool with three legs, and diet and exercise are only two of the legs. Most of us don't work on the third leg, which supports the other two.

And that third leg is the rest of your life. Without it, the diet and exercise programs rarely work.

So here's something you can do to support the rest of your life and to make the diet and exercise program more complete: ask four questions.

1) What did you accomplish yesterday?
2) Why is that important to you?
3) What further progress could you make in that area of your life?
4) What specific action could you take to further your progress?

These questions promote self-awareness, consciousness and mindfulness, and will help you gain strength and perspective on everything else you're doing. The few moments of reflection needed to answer them will produce countless dividends in the rest of your life, including by the way, your weight loss program.

These questions help you focus on what's important to you, and the answers help you make minor "course corrections" in the trajectory of your life. You'll find them a powerful tool that can help you achieve your goals, live your vision, and gain personal power in the process.

Do them every day for a month.

Then watch what happens.

Enjoy the journey.

* *(with gratitude and acknowledgement to my friend, Jack Canfield)*

8 WAYS TO BREAK A PLATEAU

You're losing weight at a nice clip when all of a sudden the scale stops moving. And it seems like there's nothing in the world you can do about it. Weeks go by and the needle hasn't budged. You've hit the moment every dieter dreads: a plateau.

When you're on a weight loss journey, the question isn't *whether* or not you'll hit a plateau, it's *when*. Plateaus are like bad weather on a long hike: it's inevitable that you'll run into it, but knowing that in advance doesn't make it one bit less frustrating or annoying when it happens. However, cheer up. Because plateaus are as common as rain, we have a pretty good idea what to do about them. There's an excellent chance that at least one of the following techniques will help you break through.

1. **Be a calorie detective**: When clients tell me they've stopped losing weight, the first thing I ask is this: *how many calories a day are you eating?* While calories are not the whole story- far from it- they are still an important component of weight loss, and they have a way of creeping up while we're not paying attention. Be brutally honest with

yourself- what are you eating and how much? Using a food diary for a while is a great way to monitor this. And yes, sodas and alcoholic beverages count! Good rule of thumb: for weight loss, aim for calories close to your target weight times.

2. **Change it up**: The classic advice when you're not making gains in an exercise program is to change your routine. Same holds true here. Low carbers might try a higher carb diet for a few days, high carbers might switch to Atkins or South Beach. At the very least, vary your ratio of protein to fat to carbs. Even varying calorie intake may have a positive effect: if you're average intake is 1500 calories try dropping to 1200 for a day, going up to 2000 and then dropping back to 1500. You get the idea- your body's gotten comfortable. It's time to   shake   things   up.

3. **Exercise a temporary ban**: Food sensitivities can cause us to hold on to weight and bloat, and the frustrating thing is that most of us don't always know which foods cause us to do this. So play the odds: highest on the list of "usual suspects" are *grains* (wheat in particular), *dairy* and *sugar*. Put a temporary ban on all three and see what happens.

4. **Kick it up a notch. Or three**: There's been a lot of rumble in the exercise community over the best way to work out for fat loss and the consensus is moving towards high intensity intervals. Forget the "fat burning zone" and go for broke. High intensity intervals- 30 to 60 seconds- are the wave of the future. If you're used to going at level three, ramp it up to level 6 for a minute then slow back down, catch your breath and do it again. Ever see

a sprinter with love handles? Training like a sprinter will lower your body fat faster than any technique I know of, plus it'll boost your metabolism and lower your weight. Bye bye plateau.

5. **Revisit strength training**: If you're not strength training, start now. And if you are, ramp it up a notch. Muscle is your greatest ally in breaking a plateau. Unfortunately many women train with weights too light to produce the metabolic boost we're looking for. Don't be afraid of heavier weights- you should reach the point where you can't do another rep sometime between reps 8-12.

6. **Up your protein**: Study after study shows that a higher ratio of protein to carbs makes losing body fat easier. Protein boosts the metabolism (in one study as much as 100 percent for 24 hours), and it also increases satiety, making it more likely that you won't overeat. A higher protein diet could be just what you need to break that plateau.

7. **Try a gentle detox**: While fasting for weight loss unsupervised is a really bad idea, the idea of giving your system a rest makes sense. One way to do it is with a "smart fast" of nothing but fruits and vegetables for a couple of days. The added fiber is always helpful, and the massive amount of nutrients and phytochemicals is like "spring cleaning" for your metabolism.

8. **Do a personal inventory**: Believe it or not, other things besides diet and exercise could be stalling your weight loss. Stress, for example. Or lack of sleep. Or medications. Take a look and see what else is going on in your life that might need

attention. Sometimes when you clean up the problems in one area of your life, problems in other areas just naturally take care of themselves.

THE ASPARTAME CONTROVERSY

Years ago, when I was growing up, my father used to regularly repeat the following mantra of parental wisdom, common among parents of baby boomers like myself: "There are two things you never discuss in public", he'd say. "Religion, and politics".

The reasoning, in that pre-Oprah time, was that bringing up either of these two subjects in conversation could virtually guarantee a heated discussion, possibly destroy friendships and at the very least, ruin an evening.

Well religion and politics are no longer forbidden topics for friendly discourse, but among nutrition experts there are still a few subjects that pretty much assure the kind of messy passion considered so gauche in my parents' time. And making anyone's top five list for an knock-down drag-out argument is the subject of artificial sweeteners.

Ask members of the food establishment, and they'll tell you, often with a sneer, that there's no scientific evidence that artificial sweeteners- specifically aspartame, the ingredient in "Equal"- causes any problems (except for people with a fairly uncommon metabolic abnormality called PPK). Perfectly safe, they say. The FDA said so. Drink diet sodas rather than regular ones, and sweeten your coffee all you like. It will help you lose weight because you'll be saving all those calories that you would be otherwise consuming in sugar. All those silly rumors of problems are just that- wild unsubstantiated rumors with no "scientific" backing. Probably started by Communists.

I'm not so sure.

Aspartame is a molecule made by joining two amino acids together, which makes it a protein fragment. That protein molecule is broken down into formaldehyde, a known carcinogen, and methanol (wood alcohol), which is a toxin capable of causing blindness. The FDA decided that this wasn't much of an issue, since the *amounts* of these two substances generated from the breakdown of aspartame didn't reach toxic levels- hence the consumer had nothing to worry about. Believe them? Well, then you have more faith in your government agencies than I do. I've met more than one person who routinely consumes a dozen cans of diet soda a day, not to mention low-fat or sugar-free deserts (which are filled with the stuff) and even if the FDA were right in thinking that small amounts of the two neurotoxins made from aspartame are "safe", I'm not sure anyone knows the long term effects of the kind of consumption we are seeing today.

The tiny protein fragment that is aspartame is able to enter the bloodstream and eventually make its way to a place in the brain called the "bare area". Now Nature, in her infinite wisdom, wisely surrounded the brain with a protective shield called the "blood-brain" barrier, meant to guard our delicate brain tissue from any undesirable riff-raff that might be circulating in the bloodstream. But in that "bare area" there's a "break" in the "gate", and it's possible for unwanted substances to enter and do some mischief. Once inside, they may stimulate the brain in an undesirable way, causing an effect called excitotoxicity. This is exactly how aspartame, and other molecules- like MSG- can theoretically present a serious problem. This point of view has been brilliantly explained and the arguments for it very well elucidated by Russell L. Blaylock, M.D., in his excellent book "Excitotoxins: The Taste That Kills". It is also a little-reported fact that aspartame accounts for somewhere around 75% of complaints about food ingredients made by consumers to the FDA.

Moving right along.

In an excellent review article in the January 2000 issue of the *Townsend Newsletter for Doctors and Patients*, Dr. H. J. Roberts chronicles his own extensive experience with the "many serious side effects and medical/public health hazards attributable to aspartame products" (his words, not mine). He believes, based on his database of over 12,000 "aspartame reactors" that aspartame can cause neurologic, psychologic, endocrine and metabolic problems, can cause, aggravate or accelerate migraine, and, in sensitive people, can be downright addictive. My friends Drs. Mike and Mary Dan Eades add that in susceptible people, "consuming aspartame may result in such symptoms as mood disturbances, sleep disturbances, headaches, dizziness, short-term memory loss, fuzzy thinking, and inability to concentrate".

For those who continue to insist, along with the FDA, that there is "no scientific evidence" for a problem, I'd like to say one word to you: cigarettes. The connection between lung cancer and cigarettes was pretty much common knowledge for almost fifteen years before the FDA finally decided there was enough evidence to put a warning label on cancer sticks. And the history of nutrition is filled with a huge gap between the discovery of something by pioneers and it's widespread acceptance by the powers that be (example: vitamin C as a cure for scurvy). Just some food for thought..

Aside from the health concerns, the funny thing is this: artificial sweeteners don't even really help you lose weight. They continue to feed your sweet tooth, making you want more sweet stuff, and lessening the chance that you will eventually stop craving sugar. And some research has shown that when people eat what they think is low-fat or low-calorie food, they "make up" for it by eating more of the "wrong" things later in the day.

Breaking the sweetener habit may not be so easy, so I recommend that if you must sweeten, do it infrequently-and when you do, use tiny amounts of the best, richest, darkest honey you can find, or, alternately, a high-quality real (not imitation) maple syrup. You can also use a wonderful herb called stevia, found in health food stores, but watch the amounts- unless you use just a little, it can have a bitter aftertaste. I'm also a huge fan of Xylitol, a sugar alcohol with some health benefits (like helping to prevent bacteria from adhering to the mucous membranes) and erythritol, (sold under the brand name TruVia). Erythritol is a sugar alcohol with virtually no impact on blood sugar and exactly zero negatives.

The good side of dumping your artificial sweetener habit is that you will probably drink less diet sodas and eat less "no-cal" deserts. Even if there was no other benefit to kicking the artificial sweetener habit, that alone would be worth the effort.

AFFORDABLE NUTRITION

There's no getting around it. The ugly truth is, it costs more to eat well than it does to eat junk.

Let's first understand why. In heavily populated, industrialized nations, especially those without a history and tradition of loving and respecting food, food is just another "product". The manufacturers of food products, like producers of other mass market goods, need to make a product that meets three conditions in order for it to be profitable: 1) it has to reach a wide market 2) it has to have a long shelf life and 3) it has to be relatively inexpensive to produce. Add to this, of course, that it has to taste and look good enough for you to want to buy it.

Notice that being of high nutritional value doesn't make the short list.

The first three of these conditions are very related. To reach a wide market, food has to travel well. That means the food has to be able to resist spoiling during the artificially long time it's asked to "remain fresh", i.e. during processing, packaging, shipping, and sitting around on the grocers shelf waiting for you to buy it. That translates to lots of preservatives and chemicals. To have a long shelf life, food has to be relatively non-perishable. That means removing, through refining, everything that would cause it to "spoil", which, coincidentally, are often the very things that makes it nutritionally useful. And to be economical to produce, it has to be resistant to annoying little problems like weather, climate, pests, bugs and the like. And that means pesticides.

And then there are the finishing touches. To make the product palatable, the food industry sweetens it. To make it visually pleasant, they color it. To make it inexpensive, they spray, genetically alter, selectively breed, mass produce, process and package crops, meat, grains and dairy into "food products" that bear about as much resemblance to what was grown on the Pilgrim's farms as Super Mario does to a backyard game of catch.

What we, the consumers, get for selling our nutritional soul is two things: convenience and price. The problem is, it's a devil's bargain. When you realize that there is a strong nutritional component to about seven out of the ten leading causes of death in this country, and that nutritional inadequacies have been linked to everything from ADD to infertility to cancer to heart disease to diabetes- (and I'm just getting started)- only then do you begin to think that this trade-off might not be such a bargain after all.

But, since we *do* live on this planet, and since we *do* need to learn to deal with things the way they are right now, what can we actually do to improve our nutritional lives without breaking the bank?

I've come up with my own top-ten list. Some of the items on it are whimsical and philosophical, and some are concrete, but all are important.

1. Realize that the biggest mistake we make as consumers is to assume that the companies producing food products have the slightest interest in our nutritional needs. "Shelf-life" is not synonymous with "Your Life"

2. Whenever possible, buy fruits and vegetables that are locally grown and produced. If you live in a big city, try to visit the farmers market. If you live in the country, try to find local suppliers.

3. Realize that food product "bargains" may not be bargains at all. Longer shelf life translates into cheaper prices, but at what cost?

4. Prepare in advance. When I say it costs more to eat healthily, I don't just mean money. Convenience and time-saving is a big part of the equation. You can even the odds against you by preparing food in advance and taking them with you.

5. Shop more often for perishables. This costs you more time, true, but the payoff is a big one. The nutrition that's lost in fruits and vegetables just by sitting around would astonish you. It doesn't cost any more to buy this stuff fresh than it does old.

6. Frozen entrees are no bargain. Believe it or not, you can buy a couple of fresh vegetables, put a little butter on them and broil some lean meat or fish for about the same cost as a frozen dinner.

7. The less processing the better. Think Caveman. Things that could be plucked, picked or grown are usually nutritional bargains, and pretty easy to find and prepare.

8. Buy organic whenever possible. I know it's more expensive, but if you can do it, it's worth it. If you have to choose, my personal candidates for most important are eggs (for the omega-3 fats) and meats (free range, antibiotic/steroid free).

9. For snacks, think nuts. It's important that they not be rancid, so get as fresh as you can, preferably raw, preferably organic. They're filling, delicious, and beat the pants off anything in the office snack machine.

10. Reprioritize. You may have to put a little more time, or in some cases, a little more money, into food. This is accomplishable only if there is a real shift in consciousness about what's important. Remember, having *less* of the really good stuff is a lot better than having *more* of junk.

Just like in life.

Affordable nutrition is probably not as cheap as we would like, but it also isn't as expensive as we think.

The question that has to be asked when it comes to buying and eating *real* food for you and your family is not "how am I gonna do it?"

It's "can I afford *not* to?"

5 BEST FOODS TO FUEL YOUR WORKOUT

Before we begin, there's one thing you need to know: The best food to eat before a workout depends on *when* you're going to eat it.

Let's say you're an early morning riser who goes to the gym on the way to work. You don't have enough time between leaving home and arriving at the gym to really digest a full breakfast, so your pre-workout snack is going to have to be really light. On the other hand, if you're working out in the middle of the afternoon, your workout is going to be fueled by your choices at lunch and you'll have a couple of hours to digest your food before hitting the gym. That means a very different "pre-workout" meal than the one you might choose if you were scrounging around the kitchen at 5:30 AM on the way to the track.

So the rule of thumb is this: the shorter the time to the workout, the less you should eat. This makes sense: it takes time to digest food, so you don't want to scarf down a huge breakfast right before getting on the treadmill. Those planning to run the marathon on Sunday usually eat a huge dinner on Saturday night. But those planning to go for a three mile jog at 5:30 AM may be fine with just an orange eaten about 20 minutes before gym time.

With that in mind, I've prepared a list of my five favorite "all around" pre-workout snacks. These work just fine whether you're an early morning exerciser and need something light, or if you're about to head out for a workout in the late afternoon and are just looking for a little extra energy to combat the "3 PM Crash".

1. **"With a Smear"**. This is one of my favorite snacks, period. I take some hearts of celery and fill in the groove with some organic almond butter or peanut butter. This snack really travels well in tuperware, and makes a terrific pre-workout snack. Why? The celery has fiber and nutrients (including calcium and vitamin A) and a ridiculously low 6 calories per medium stalk. The nut butter has protein and fat. The overall calories are low and this really fills you up without slowing you down. Great "slow-release" energy for a terrific workout.

2. **"The Double A"**: An apple with almonds. The apple is the perfect food for a preworkout snack. It's sugar load is very moderate, it contains valuable pectin fiber which slows the entrance of that sugar into the bloodstream, and it's a nutritional powerhouse containing vitamins and minerals and antioxidants. Combine it with about a dozen almonds, which adds some fat and protein, further slows the entrance of the sugar into the bloodstream for sustained energy, and keeps hunger away.

3. **"Whey to go"**: Whey protein is my favorite kind of protein powder. Not only is it extremely high quality, bioavailable protein, but it supports the immune system by providing the body with the building blocks for glutathione, arguably the body's most important antioxidant. And studies

indicate that whey protein may boost weight-loss efforts. According to one French study, consuming whey before exercise supports fat burning and may help with gaining or maintaining lean body mass. I suggest a whey protein shake made with either water alone or with frozen berries. The berries add fiber, nutrients, some extra carbohydrates, and make for a more delicious drink.

4. **"Berry Cheesy"**: Here's a little tidbit of info that you might enjoy: In my book, "The 150 Healthiest Foods on the Planet" I asked 16 of the best known experts in the country to contribute their personal "top ten" list of favorite healthy foods. Berries- especially blueberries- made the list of more experts than any other food. Berries are loaded with phytonutrients, antioxidants and fiber, and are low in sugar. Mix a bowl of berries with a piece of string cheese for the perfect pre-workout snack. The string cheese has 8 grams of protein, some fat to keep hunger at bay, and only about 80 calories. Plus it's an excellent source of calcium.

5. **"TG/ Too Good"**: The initials of this snack stand for turkey and grapes. It's a perfectly matched trifecta of protein, carbs and low-calories to take the edge off your hunger and prime your exercise pump. Four small slices of deli packaged turkey contain only 87 calories but give you more than 14 grams of protein, plus some of the cancer-fighting mineral selenium to boot. A cup of grapes adds some carbs to the mix together with all the health-giving phytochemicals grapes are known for. Suggestion: Go for fresh turkey whenever possible as the packaged kind is high in sodium, and go for red or purple grapes as they have a

higher antioxidant content.

Obviously there are other choices besides my five favorites. In a pinch, I'll use a protein bar, though you'll want to watch the sugar content and look out for the presence of trans-fatty acids. One of my favorites is Atkins Advantage, though there are others you may like as well. And hard boiled eggs are another secret weapon in the search for portable protein that combines nicely with a little fruit (like an apple).

Also remember: what you eat after the workout is even more important than what you eat before it. That's when your muscles are hungry and your depleted stores of glycogen (muscle sugar) need replacing. The "golden hour" after the workout is the time when those muscles soak up nutrients most effectively. Choose what you eat after the workout with just as much care as you choose that pre-workout snack!

CRITIQUING YOUR INNER CRITIC

Last night I met a young actress friend of mine named Lynn for drinks. She had just returned from L.A. where she had filmed her first episode of a new series. I asked her how it went.

"Well", she said, unenthusiastically, "it was OK I guess".

"You don't sound too happy about it" I commented.

"Well, I could've done better. I was a little nervous, and I rushed my lines. I didn't breathe enough. I didn't take chances. I played it safe. I think I made the character dull".

"Go on"

"You know they said it was great, but I have all these voices in my head telling me what was wrong with it, and then I start worrying that maybe they didn't really like me, and maybe they'll replace me with another actress, and everyone will know I'm really not all that talented.."

Now interestingly, I have another actor friend who

works on the same show. Shortly after the day in question, he had called me and said "Man, Lynn did great on her first day! Everyone loves her. She blew everyone away with her performance!".

So much for the impact of reality on our inner voices.

"I know, I know what you're going to say" Lynn continued. "I'm being too critical. I shouldn't be saying all these negative things about my performance, I should just think positive thoughts".

Actually, I said, that's not at all what I was going to say.

What I was going to say was this: your inner critic needs a little work.

See, those inner voices of ours serve a function. Without them, we have no way of evaluating our actions or our productivity. The inner critic provides us with a terrific feedback mechanism, kind of like a navigational system on an airplane. It lets us know if we are on course; if we are off course, it tells us by how much so that we can correct the flight plan. Turning it off deprives us of a unique opportunity.

What I said to my friend was this: OK, we've heard what your critic had to say. Now let's see if we can critique the critic. Teachers learn to teach by being critiqued by other teachers; coaches learn to coach by being coached on the art of coaching. The trick here isn't to silence your inner critic, I told my friend.

The trick here is to make him more effective.

So let's apply this to weight loss.

Let's say you've been really sticking to your program. You've been eating well, staying on course, keeping away from trigger foods, and seeing real progress. You're invited to a wedding. You get there with the best intentions, but, after all, it's a special occasion, you have a glass of wine, someone talks you into sampling one of the scrumptious little pastry appetizers, and in a New York minute it seems you've downed about 4,000 excess calories of every food that you've managed to keep away from in the last six weeks.

Look, everyone on the planet has done this at one time or another. Let's put that fact aside for the moment. What I'm interested in right now is not *whether* it happens, but what you do when it does.

I want to know if your "inner critic" is doing his job well. Is he helping you? or is he beating you up?

How much damage has the person downing those 4,000 calories really done? In reality, not much. Maybe a pound or two, tops, which can easily be dropped over the next few days. The real damage comes when the inner voices get the microphone.

Most of my clients, after "blowing" a food plan in an incident like this, report that they go through very predictable inner dialogues. You probably know what this dialogue is. How deeply into the abyss of this particular dialogue you happen to journey depends on a lot of factors, but I'm willing to bet some form of the following litany is not exactly unfamiliar ground. Here goes:

"Well, there goes the diet. I might as well eat all of it. It doesn't matter, since I'll never be able to stick to anything. I'll never have any discipline. I'll never get this weight off. I was just kidding myself. I'm a big loser"

Now let's coach that little inner voice we just heard speak.

First, some questions.

Did the voice make you feel inspired? Make you feel encouraged? After listening to it, did you feel like a winner? Did it play to your strong points while pointing out where you needed work?

Did you learn anything from it?

If not, your inner critic has some work to do.

Here's what I told my actress friend: How much better would it have been, in terms of your future work and your well-being, if your inner "coach" had said: "Hey, good job. Little nervous, but that's to be expected. But it's OK, cause it gave your performance a bit of an edge. Next time breathe more. You've got great instincts.. trust them. Next time, take a little more risk".

That's good coaching.

How much better would it be if you said to yourself, on the day after the wedding, "Hey, it was a special occasion... I did what I did. It's no big deal. Look at where I've come from and how much I've accomplished. I'm in charge here, and I choose to get right back on track. I haven't lost that much ground, and in the scheme of things, it doesn't mean anything. A week from now it'll be forgotten. I had fun and it's done. Cool. Let's move on".

Here's your homework. Next time your inner critic starts mouthing off, let him have his say. (He'll have it whether you like it or not).

Then give him some coaching on how he could do his job better.

After all, the better he is, the better you'll be.

AIRPORT EATING

This article is for anyone who ever spent time in an airport.

I spend a lot of time in airports. This results in the development of much useful knowledge. For example, I know exactly where to find the National Enquirer in virtually every Hudson News store in America. I can tell you exactly what color travel pillows they have at Brookstone's. I know what rap CD is on special at AirTunes.

And, out of necessity, I've also learned where to find actual food in airports.

Which is no easy task, thank you very much.

But, as they say, what doesn't kill you makes you stronger, and the experience has made me something of an expert on eating on the road.

Now you don't have to spend a lot of time in airports to benefit from my experience. This article is actually for anyone who travels. Or orders take-out. Or goes out to dinner. Or has a social life. Or a business life. Come to think of it, it's for anyone who has a life period.

In today's world, few folks have the luxury of eating all their meals at an actual table, let alone at home. If you live in a big city, the sight of folks rushing through the streets, chomping furiously on anything they can hold in one hand, signaling for a taxi with the other, is old hat to you. You've got kids to chauffeur around, schedules to meet, meetings to go to, games to cheer at, ballet class, the gym, board meetings that last all afternoon, committees to chair and families to spend time with. You're constantly in motion. The days of Esther dropping by Lucy's for coffee to break up the morning monotony are long over. Morning monotony? Are you kidding? For better or worse, we live a Tasmanian devil of an existence that's exciting, maddening and frustrating all at the same time, and for those of us trying to eat well, a veritable minefield of potential disaster.

I know. I'm the one who lives in airports.

To make matters as bad as they could be, there seems to be an unwritten law which I call "Bowden's law of inverse quality". It states that the quality of food goes down as portability and accessibility go up. There ain't no organic fruits and vegetables at the food court, folks. The airports are filled with crummy, sugar-laden "pick me up" treats, the take-out counters filled with bad, processed meat and deli food, and business travelers are well aware that even the best hotel restaurants are a cornucopia of temptation, made all the worse by the fact that by the time we sit down to dinner we're starving and not even the basket that the bread comes in is safe from us.

So what to do? Unless you've got access to a time machine, eating on the run- or at least on the move- is likely to remain a fact of life. The opportunity here is to become a master of your circumstances rather than a victim of them.

Here are my top ten tips for how to do just that:

1) **Think proactive**. Most of the trouble comes from waiting till you're in the middle of an emergency hunger situation before taking action (like being without food all afternoon and coming face to face with a convenient snack machine). A little planning goes a long way. If you know you're gonna be stuck in a meeting, take along something you can eat quickly and discreetly that will keep your blood sugar from plummeting and your cravings at bay. Best choices: Celery sticks and a small container of peanut butter for dipping. String cheese and an apple. Nuts--(but watch the quantity). And the best health food in the world: A can of sardines!

2) **Use lettuce instead of bread**. You can wrap some leftover chicken in a lettuce leaf and eat it in the car or anywhere else a sandwich would work. Throw on some tomatoes and a drizzle of olive oil and you've got a decent mini-meal. Some fast food restaurants are now offering their burgers made exactly this way.

3) **Find healthy food that travels well**. Top tips: Cottage cheese, yogurt, celery, peppers, carrots, and apples. Throw some berries into a Tupperware with some cottage cheese and nuts and take it with you. In a pinch, high-protein low-carb snack bars beat the pants of standard machine food.

4) **Prepare the food before**. (This is the corollary

of "think proactively"). Bake a week's worth of sweet potatoes on a Sunday, cut 'em in half and take them with you as snacks during the week. They're as portable as you can get, they taste great cold, and they are loaded with vitamins.

5) **Think nuts**. Here's what they do: provide good fats, fiber, minerals and a little protein. They also fill you up. The key is to not buy the big bags and nibble all day. Make your own little sandwich bags with a dozen or so nuts in each, and combine them with an apple or some string cheese. Best choices: walnuts, pecans and almonds.

6) **Think unusual foods**. Paleolithic man carried around the original energy bar called Pemmican. It's made with pressed grass fed meat sweetened with dried cherries. You can get them through a link on my website. It tastes way better than it sounds, and it's healthy as can be!

7) **Find the chicken Caesar**. At long last this has become a staple of take-out restaurants in airports. Trust me, I know. Buy them!

8) **Know how to order in a restaurant**. When eating out, choose fish, lean meat or chicken, and a ton of vegetables. Tell them to hold the potatoes or rice and double the veggies. Send the bread back, and skip dessert (or order fresh berries, even if they're not on the menu).

With a little thinking ahead, meals on the road don't have to be a disaster. And the challenge of eating well can actually be fun. Just ask me. I'm the one snacking on nuts in the Jet Blue Terminal.

FOOD OVERDOSE

A couple of weeks ago I was invited to my friend Billy's annual Christmas eve party. Billy recently adopted a border terrier, named Ivy, to whom I promptly became a godparent. (Dog people will understand, don't worry if you don't....)

Anyway, I get to the party, and I notice something peculiar about little Ivy. She has trouble jumping up into my lap without assistance, which is something she always does effortlessly when I see her. She is moving about the crowded room rather slowly. In fact, if I didn't know better, I'd say she appeared to be almost staggering. When she finally *does* struggle up into my lap, she promptly falls asleep.

"What's up with the dog?", I ask Billy's partner, Doug. Smilingly, he responds.

"Why, it's simple", he says, stroking the puppy's distended little belly.

"She's food drunk".

Now what's interesting is that every time I've told this

story, virtually everyone in earshot nods knowingly, even though they may never have heard the term before.

Food drunk. The dog, normally a completely fearless, animated little energizer battery that could have been the "before" model in the old Saturday Night Live bit about "doggie uppers" was disoriented, sluggish, sleepy and… well, drunk.

Sound familiar?

See, in the wild, a dog like Ivy knows exactly what it's meant to eat. Her canine ancestors scavenged for food, just like ours did, and over eons of time learned what was "good" for them and what wasn't; they learned to avoid that which was poisonous, and to seek out that which was nurturing. If they didn't learn that lesson, they died, and their survivors presumably had better instincts for being smart about what to eat. In other words, they learned to know what their bodies needed.

Who could predict what would happen when you let an adorable terrier loose in a Manhattan cocktail party full of Christmas revelers who can't resist feeding it everything from chocolate covered peanuts, to homemade cakes to cheese balls to cold cuts to Rex's homemade brownies and every other hors d'oeuvre it appreciatively gobbles up as we all smile and say how cute it is.

We've all been Ivy.

And we've all been "food drunk". Only more often than not, we call it "bingeing".

Food is powerful medicine. It has the ability to affect our mood, our energy, our sense of aliveness, our strength and our endurance. And, like medicine, the wrong kind in the wrong amounts can…well, if not kill you, at the very least ruin your day.

Not to mention your self-esteem.

Like our canine brethren (dog lovers will understand and forgive the technically wrong use of the word), we too evolved from hunter-gatherer societies where we learned to understand what our bodies needed. Furthermore, nature co-operated. It put in our path what we were designed to "run best" on. The emergence of the "Paleolithic diet" as one of the hottest research and discussion topics in current nutritional thinking bears testimony to the importance of this concept. And what we were meant to "run best" on was some combination of what grew, was plucked, could be gathered, hunted or fished for. We knew intuitively how much or how little to eat, because we *needed* to know that to survive.

I don't think Nature anticipated the Christmas office party. Or the wedding buffet.

Nor the modern day supermarket.

Confronted with choices that are so stunningly diverse-- packaged, manufactured "food products" that bear little resemblance to anything like "live foods"-- surrounded with modern day supermarkets which offer all of these conveniently, instantly and usually round-the-clock, many of us do what Ivy did at the Christmas party.

We overdose.

And because we can no longer count on our environment to co-operate with us by putting in our paths only wholesome, nutritious foods that let our bodies burn the food equivalent of "clean energy", we have to make a substantial effort to get back on track. The constant exposure and easy access to a stupendously obscene amount of the wrong kinds of foods makes it harder and harder to rely on what our bodies "tell" us. When the caveman craved sweets, it meant he needed to climb the nearest tree to pick a fruit that was rich in vitamin C. When we crave sweets, it means eat a Twinkie.

That's why diets *do* sometimes work. We've become so acclimated to doing what our bodies *want*, rather than what they *need*, that we can no longer tell the difference. Diets provide structure, and structure can often be the path to re-education.

When you want to kick a drug habit, there's ultimately only one way to do it. You need to do whatever it takes to really understand what your body feels like and functions like "clean", without the drug.

Does that mean you can never have a fun Christmas eve like Ivy did?

No. But it *does* mean that, like Ivy, you'll be a lot happier puppy if you eat the foods that nature intended for you.

7 TIPS FOR HOLIDAY EATING

Wonderful as they may be for everything else, when it comes to sticking to a weight loss plan, holidays can be downright deadly.

Since holiday eating can mean so many things- family stuff, office parties, special desserts, the inevitable boxes of cookies at the office water cooler- it's hard to come up with one sure-fire strategy that will work for everyone in all situations.

There is, however, one strategy you can use that will invariably make a difference no matter what the particulars of the situation. And it can be summed up in one word:

Rehearsal.

Most of us know what we're going up against in situations where we've previously encountered trouble. For some it's the sight of the Thanksgiving table and relatives you haven't seen all year. For others, it's virtually everyone in the office bringing in their aunt's special Christmas cookies. For still others it's the stress eating associated with the mixed emotions of family reunions and juggling even more commitments than the usual overload. Even vacations can be stressful, and if they happen to involve airports at holiday time, fuggedaboudit.

Add it all up and you've got a potential disaster. You're looking at emotional and physical overload, and what that means for your waistline (let alone your sense of well-being) is not good.

Rehearsing a problem situation in your mind *before* it happens helps you to arm yourself with strategies, visualize yourself doing them, and experience the positive results. That way you're not caught unprepared, and you can actually practice reacting to a variety of dangerous situations.

Rehearsal is what coaches do with their athletes; it's what boxing trainers do with their fighters. "When he throws that left hook, you step in under and throw a right to the body", says the coach, basically "rehearsing" the moves his athlete will make using visualization and planning. Studies have shown improvement in sports performance just by doing visualization exercises. Basketball players who mentally rehearse shots perform better than those who don't; pianists who spend 30 minutes mentally rehearsing a passage perform that passage almost as well as they would if they had actually physically practiced it.

You can do the same thing with the holidays.

Of course to do this effectively, you have to be clear on what you want to happen. That's why I like using a tool I call the "proactive food journal". Here's how to do it: Pick a day, visualize what it's going to be like, where you're going to be and with whom. Think about what food is likely to be available. When you're likely to be hungry. What the circumstances are going to be.

Is your Aunt Tina going to be there insisting you try her special key lime pie? Are you going to be in a restaurant known for its crème brulee and homemade breads? Are you going to be in a fast-food restaurant taking care of six kids? Is your sister that you hate going to be there watching everything you eat and sitting in silent judgment?

Now write down what you're going to eat. Decide in advance, and decide early in the day, or the night before. Visualize the situation. If there's temptation or anxiety, close your eyes and picture it. Hear in your mind's ear what people will say. See yourself responding in a way that would make you proud of yourself, whatever that is. It might mean allowing yourself one or two bites of something "off your diet", it might mean being spartan. The point here is not *what* you choose, but *that* you choose it.

And that you then stick to it.

As Sondheim wrote, "The choice may have been mistaken. The choosing was not". The point here is to put *you* in charge of what happens, not the circumstances.

If you can accomplish that, you have begun a journey that will not only help you manage your weight, but will empower you in all areas of your life.

Here are 7 of my favorite tips on how to use visualization to help you with holiday eating:

1. Close your eyes and picture the situation clearly.
2. Ask yourself whether what's being offered is going to be something that supports you in what you're doing or takes you off course.
3. Decide what you wish to allow yourself to indulge

in- if anything- and when you decide to do it, indulge in it with gusto.

4. Make the choice and take the action.

5. Don't arrive hungry. A cup of soup or vegetable juice before arriving at a big event will help keep you in charge of your own actions.

6. Remember that stress leads to stress eating. Stress management is a critical part of managing weight gain during the holiday season!

7. If you do indulge, for goodness sake enjoy it!

FOOD AND LOVE

OK let's face it. When you were a little baby, and things didn't go well, and you needed comfort and love, your mother didn't bring you a plate of asparagus.

From before you can remember, deep in the DNA of your unconsciousness, food has always been conditioned to some amalgamation of love, security, safety and/or comfort.

It begins with milk- the real kind, not the fake kind you get in the supermarket. It had more fat than the bottled kind, less protein, and was warm and sweet to your infant taste buds- in short, it was exactly what your body needed, and it soothed the pain of hunger. Plus, since it didn't just materialize from the sky, its delivery usually meant that someone who cared about you was around to provide it. A nice double whammy in the conditioning department.

Bingo. Home run. An association embedded in your cortex, a Pavlovian field demonstration, and an equation is forever formed: food equals love.

And boy, did you learn that lesson well.

And, in one fashion or another, it's probably always been this way. No matter how much we evolved over the past few million years, one truth remains: the human infant has one of the longest periods of helplessness of any mammal. Without a caretaker, it won't survive. This serves a double evolutionary purpose- not only does it bond the infant to the mother, but it bonds the caretaker to the cared for. It is the building-block molecule of the social contract, and without it, bad stuff happens.

Fast forward twenty to eighty years from the cradle. You feel pain. You feel loneliness. You feel frustration. You feel empty. What do you reach for?

I'll give you a hint. It's not broccoli.

Food and love have been celebrated and ritualized in one way or another for as long as there has been community. Holiday meals. Wedding banquets. Dinner dates. Family gatherings. "*Eat*, Darling!" Birthday parties. Tribal hunts and subsequent feasts. Celebration of the Mass. Passover. You name it, if there is social meaning to it, there's going to be food involved.

Here's a quick test. I'll tell you a phrase, you tell me what you think of first. Ready?

Valentine's Day.

Let me guess. It wasn't broccoli.

So here we are, confronted with one of the great temptations of civilized life, another holiday that is completely, irrevocably, unalterably linked with love, chocolate, sweetness and romance.

What to do, what to do…

It seems downright Scrooge-like to call in the food police at this time. So no, I'm not going to do that. I mean, look, I ate cake at my wedding, and I'll probably down a couple of creamy little Godivas come February 14th. I'm hardly above temptation. Recreational eating is one of the joys of life. No one ever suggested that you never bite into a chocolate again, or enjoy a creamy luxurious ice-cream cake, or taste a superbly made French dessert while on vacation.

But the message I would like to leave you with is this: It pays off big-time to understand that primitive connection between food and love, because it's not the Valentine's Day candy that's going to do you in, and it's not the bi-annual wedding cake or Thanksgiving sweet-potato pie.

What does us in, so to speak, is the day to day habit of making ourselves feel good by giving ourselves what we *want*, rather than learning to want what we *need*.

Our inner infants didn't have to make that distinction. If all went well, what they needed and what they wanted were the same thing.

We can learn that lesson again in adulthood.

Food can still be a part of love. But how much better if it's the food that nourishes and sustains us, rather than just the food that feels good for the moment.

And how much better still if, over time, those two things can be one and the same.

7 IMPOSTERS: HEALTHY FOODS THAT AREN'T

Farm Raised Salmon: Sorry to say, there's no comparison between farm-raised salmon and the wild variety. Farm-raised salmon have up to 8 times the level of carcinogenic PCBs as wild salmon, and they're lower in omega-3 fats. Penned salmon are fed grain and fishmeal and a ton of antibiotics, and they don't have nearly as high nutritional value as their wild relatives. In addition, wild salmon get their red color from astaxanthin, a powerful antioxidant that comes from their natural food source, krill. Farmed salmon get their color from a color wheel.

Most supermarket cereals: With few exceptions, most supermarket cereals are fiber lightweights. The overwhelming majority are loaded with sugar. Most have a very high glycemic impact, meaning they raise blood sugar quickly, contributing to mood swings and energy dips. Whole grains are better, but those who are sensitive to blood sugar fluctuations will have still have to be careful. The best cereals are old-fashioned oatmeal, and a few standouts like Fiber One and All-Bran. Most of the others- not so good. Look for those that pass the "5 and 5" rule: less than 5 grams of sugar, more than 5 grams of fiber.

Granola bars: Candy bars masquerading as a health food. While some "energy" or "protein" bars are the genuine article, most are simply chewy versions of candy bars, with very little fiber, lots of processed carbs, and a ton of sugar. You're better off "rolling your own" out of raw oats, chopped almonds, coconut flakes, raisins and a dollop of raw organic honey.

Frozen yogurt: Frozen yogurt is a prime example of the triumph of marketing over good sense. The only thing frozen yogurt has in common with real yogurt is that they're both white. Real yogurt- one of the most healthy foods on earth-- is loaded with live cultures which support your digestive health. The live culture content of frozen yogurt is precisely zero. What's more, frozen yogurt is usually filled with chemicals, and the artificial sweeteners in the non-fat kind can cause cravings just like sugar. You're better off with real, creamy, organic ice cream. Just don't eat too much.

Canola Oil: Sounds sacrilegious, but canola oil isn't such a health bargain after all. Conventional canola oil is processed by high temperature mechanical pressing. It goes through caustic refining, bleaching and degumming. The high temperatures needed to extract the oil from the rapeseed plant make it's highly touted omega-3's rancid and foul smelling, requiring them to be deodorized, a process which creates some trans-fatty acids. Unless it's cold-pressed and organic, stay away.

Egg white omelets: OK, these aren't exactly unhealthy, they're just utterly unnecessary. The whole concept of egg white omelets is left over from the 80's obsession with low-fat, and when it comes to eggs, it's a huge mistake. The yolk contains the superstars of eye nutrition, **lutein and xeazanthin,** which need fat to be absorbed properly. Egg yolks are an important source

phosphatidylcholine an important nutrient for brain health. And half the fat in the yolk isn't even saturated to begin with!

Apple juice: Apples- healthy. Apple juice- not so fast. One cup of apple juice has zero grams of fiber, 117 calories, and 29 grams of carbs of which 27 are sugar (and your typical serving is a lot more than a cup). Sorry, but that's not a health drink, it's sugar water with apple flavoring. The implications of giving our kids 8 cups a day of this stuff is just now beginning to be understood. An apple a day keeps the doctor away. Wish we could say the same about apple juice, but we can't.

THE ETERNAL TRUTHS
OF DIETING

The other night, I was at a party and I ran into some fitness professionals that I hadn't seen in almost a decade, not since we all shared floor space as personal trainers at the same gym in New York. After we reminisced for a while, we began talking about the different paths our lives had taken since those early days. One of the trainers was now a Pilates specialist; another was into yoga; a third was a physical therapist.

All of us had obviously matured a bit since the early days when all that mattered was muscle, muscle, muscle, and the "only" way to lose fat was a low-fat diet.

Our clients were still into looking good, of course, but health concerns had broadened their vision and expanded their concerns. The only thing that had not changed was that the vast majority of the people who came to us had issues with their weight, and all of us agreed that if we learned one lesson in our decade of experience, it was that people responded very very differently not only to exercise regimes but to dietary ones.

With that as a background, one of the trainers turned to

me and asked the following question: "You have a radio show and a column", she said. "You give advice, you interview people, you answer questions for a broad audience. But we've all agreed that people are so different, and that what's right for one might be wrong for another. Knowing that, how do you talk to a broad audience? How do you give advice that everyone can use knowing that each person is unique?"

It's a very good question, and here's the short answer: You start with the basics.

You lay out a buffet of healthy choices that have served human beings for hundreds of thousands of years, and you empower people to get to know their own unique biochemistry so that they know how much to put on their plate from this basic menu.

See, the human genus has been on this planet for a very, very long time. During most of that time, the food supply was pretty unvarnished- animals to hunt, fish to catch, things to pluck and gather. Our digestive systems are pretty much the same now as they were then- it takes a very, very long time for adaptations to occur and most nutritional anthropologists don't think our nutritional needs have changed much since we were cavemen. Agriculture didn't appear till about ten thousand years ago, a mere minute in the history of mankind. If you look at the most common food allergens, they are nearly all foods that were introduced into the human diet fairly recently - wheat, corn, dairy, soy and peanuts being perfect examples.

So with this in mind, what's good advice to give the

"average person" who wants to lose weight? Or, to put it in a bigger context, what's good advice for people who want to get healthy? Does it even make sense to lay out a "perfect" diet and expect it to work for everyone?

Obviously, the answer is no. But what *does* make sense is to lay out a simple menu of foods most likely to nourish and least likely to cause problems in the largest number of people. If you begin by laying out this basic buffet of foods that have been in the human food supply for hundreds of thousands of years, and at the same time teach people how to learn the connection between food and weight, food and mood, food and energy, food and allergy…. Well then, you've laid the groundwork for a diet that can not only help you lose fat, but can also boost your immune system, decrease symptoms of allergy and sensitivity, provide high levels of nutrients during pregnancy, and possibly extend and improve life. This groundwork can be laid with a few simple, eternal rules, and they are broad enough and general enough to work for absolutely everybody.

Start with these, and then customize to taste. If you begin here, you can't go wrong. And, like any buffet, you personally may find visiting one section of the table more than others, but that's part of the adventure of personal discovery.

SAY **YES** TO:

1. **Protein**- from organic, free range sources. Eggs from free-range chickens. Choose meats that are grass-fed and free of hormones and antibiotics.

2. **Fish, fish and more fish**. (a *specific* protein choice that should be emphasized as much as possible)

3. **Vegetables**. As fresh as possible, grown locally if possible, grown organically if possible, in season if possible. Frozen are fine. Canned are not*. Get as many colors in your basket as possible.

4. **Fruits**. Same as above. Berries are particularly good. * (There are occasional exceptions to the canned rule, but they're few and far between. Two I can think of are canned pineapple in its own juice, and canned pumpkin).

5. **Nuts and seeds**. Raw if possible. Soak nuts overnight to increase digestibility.

6. **Traditional, healthy fats**. Get a good mix of omega-3's (fish, flaxseed), omega-6 (cold pressed organic vegetable oils, evening primrose oil) and omega-9's (extra-virgin olive oil). Butter. Avocado. Coconut.

SAY **NO** TO:

1. **Processed food**. Eat as little as possible. Read labels. The more things you can't pronounce, the more possibility of problems. The longer the *shelf* life, the worse for *your* life.

2. **"Partially Hydrogenated Anything"**. You'll be surprised at how many packaged foods this applies to. Throw out your margarine. (And don't necessarily believe the "no trans fats" plastered on labels. The

FDA allows anything with less than a half a gram per "serving" to be called zero. If the ingredients read "partially hydrogenated oil", the stuff's got trans-fats no matter what the package says).

3. **"Instant Meals"**. Avoid "instant" anything. It didn't come that way in the wild.

4. **Packaged treats**. Try to avoid foods that are packaged, snacks, chips, baked "treats", crackers and fat-free cookies

5. **Sugar.** The hardest to give up completely, but if you can, you'll see the most benefits.

6. **Artificial sweeteners**. Bulletin: they don't help you lose weight.

7. **Sodas**. Of any kind (they didn't drink these in the wild either).

8. **Fried food**. Seriously.

Most people will find it difficult to eliminate grains, and many don't have to. But it's always an interesting experiment to eliminate wheat for a week or so just to see if you feel any different. Same with dairy. If there are no allergies or hypersensitivities, these can be included in the diet, but go easy on the grains. They're a recent addition to the human diet, and we eat far too many of them. Go out of your way to find *whole grains*, and try some that are gluten-free. Don't make them the main attraction of your diet if you're trying to lose weight.

These are probably as close to "universal" truths in

nutrition as we're likely to get: No one gets healthy on processed food. No one loses weight on packaged junk. No one does their health or their waistline any good with toxic meats, foods that have been fried in day old rancid oil and vats of sodas (the majority of fast food restaurants), and no one does particularly well on six servings of bread a day. Sugar = sabotage. Vegetables benefit everyone, as do the right kinds of fat and protein.

A menu like this respects the fact that everyone is different- Some people can do with more carbohydrates than others, some with more fat, some with more protein. But begin your experiment in personal empowerment with this basic, scaled down menu, and you're guaranteed to improve your health and your waistline.

You'll probably learn some interesting things about yourself at the same time.

FOOD DIARIES AND JOURNALS

Anyone who has followed what I've called "*the diet wars*" knows that the possibility of getting ten nutrition specialists to agree on anything is only slightly more likely than a mutual declaration of love between Joe Frasier and Muhammad Ali. So when just about everyone in is in agreement about some aspect of weight control or health, my ears perk up and so should yours.

We know, for example, that vegetables are in this rarefied category of "things about which there is complete agreement". What other food or supplement, you might well wonder, qualifies for this VIP status of nutritional wonder substances?

Turns out it's not a food at all.

What it is, is a food journal.

And most clinical nutritionists, whose orientations range from A (Atkins) to Z (Zone) agree that it is critical to success. Here's why:

When you keep a food diary (or more effectively, a journal), you're basically undertaking a project the sole purpose of which is to better understanding *you*. The ancients believed that "naming" something allowed you to master it, or at least to understand it better. Journaling, in a way, let's you master the universe by using the power of your own voice, albeit through the written word. In our case, the universe we're attempting to master is that of our own bodies, but the possibility exists that we wind up mastering so much more.

Disc jockeys have a saying: *play it and say it.* We journal-keepers should adopt that saying but with a twist: *Say* it, and you will *play* it. By constantly telling the truth, in the safe and private context of your own writing, you make your word law in the universe. Name it and you own it.

The journal helps you to crystallize what you're feeling and focus in on what is actually going on. Feelings are often diffuse, elusive, and hard to pinpoint. Separating "what happened" from the story we make up about it is easier when we write it down. (Think Sgt. Joe Friday in <u>*Dragnet*</u>: "Just the facts, ma'am, just the facts".) Always remember my favorite mantra: The facts don't make us miserable… the *meaning we attach to them* (our "stories") do.

"I lost out on an audition", "My boyfriend didn't call me" or "I gained ten pounds" are simple, neutral facts. Where they get us in trouble is when we begin to make them "mean" something. "*I'm a crummy actress that no one will ever hire*", or "*No man will ever find me attractive*" or "*I'm a fat slob with no will power*" are examples of the "stories" that we *make-up* about the previously mentioned facts, the "meanings" that we arbitrarily weld to them until it becomes increasingly difficult to simply say "what happened" independently from what we think it "means".

Once you truly understand the difference, you're well on the way to disempowering the self-destructive "story" and simply dealing with the truth rather the excess baggage you attach to it.

A good exercise for separating fact from personal fiction is what I call the "so what" exercise. State the "fact" that you think is upsetting you as plainly and neutrally as you can; then add the comment, "so what?" (I gained ten pounds". "so what?") "*SO WHAT*?" the little voice in your head screams. "*So I'm a big fat slob with no will power and I'll never have a life, That's "so what!!"*. But that is not "the fact" at all. The "fact" is this: you gained ten pounds. That you will "never have a life" is a *story*. The journal lets you clarify this all-important distinction, so that you can deal with the facts ("so what?") and leave the story behind. (Hint: the facts by themselves are *never* as bad as the stories you tell yourself about them).

Food journals also have the more mundane purpose of letting us really see what goes into our mouth. Unconsciousness is the biggest enemy of success in weight loss. Most overeating- in fact, most *eating*- is unconscious. It's a mindless, habitual, conditioned reaction to a wide variety of cues, few of which have to do with hunger. By forcing them into consciousness by writing down what you're doing, when you're doing it, and how you're feeling at the time, you get the unprecedented opportunity to really examine what's what and to transform "automatic" behavior into that which comes from conscious choice.

Journals also let us begin to make connections between food and mood. One of the problems with the American diet is that we eat so much, of so many things, and our physical and emotional reactions to these foods are often so delayed, that we rarely get an opportunity to actually do the detective work that would lead us to discover the effects food have on our moods, energy levels, and mental outlook. Similarly, by making room in the journal for notes about what was happening and what we were feeling, we can also bring into clear focus just what conditions are dangerous triggers for "non-nurturing" eating behaviors.

Finally, for many people, the journal is one of the only places where we can really be alone with ourselves. Freed from the knowledge that someone else will see and judge what we're feeling and saying, many of us discover that it is truly possible to explore feelings, behaviors, fantasies and even "unacceptable" thoughts that we spend a great deal of psychic energy keeping hidden, not only from our loved ones but from ourselves. The journal is your own private letter to yourself. Freed from the constraints of social acceptability and "proper behavior" you're able to really delve into the deepest parts of yourself.

In ten years of practice, I've yet to meet someone who gave journaling an honest try and didn't get some benefit out of it, often a benefit that was wholly unexpected yet profoundly impactful. The beautiful part of it is that there's no "right" way to do it. You can scrawl angry words on a page, "say" things to parents, husbands, loved ones that you've never been able to "say", or just make a simple old list of what you're eating and when.

Be willing to be surprised by the results. You almost certainly will be.

IS YOUR INNER CRITIC HOLDING YOU BACK?

A client recently came to me - let's call him Pete- who weighed in the mid 200's. Heavy most of his life, he was finally ready to do something to change his high stress, eat-on-the-run, junk-food lifestyle and begin taking care of himself. Since I no longer take on personal training clients, I worked with him on his nutrition program and sent him to the best trainer I know in New York, Bill Humphries, who put him on the remarkable "Body Attack" program.

To make a long story short, it's been about six months, and this guy, who could barely walk a flight of steps without puffing when we first met, recently ran an eight and a half minute mile on the treadmill. He's dropped 40 pounds, and looks and feels better than he ever has.

Now here's the thing.

Pete's dad had been an ex-marine, and heavily valued traditionally masculine behavior- "toughing it out", "boys don't cry", Monday night football... you get the drift. Pete's a kind of an "artsy", creative type, and felt like he could never really please his dad in the "testosterone-driven-activity" department. What's more, Pete's early attempts at sports weren't very successful, and his father teased him mercilessly for his poor performance.

On more than one occasion, his father said to him, only half-jokingly, "Man, Pete… you run like a _girl_!"

That comment, in the way that certain childhood incidents have of sticking to the flypaper of our unconscious and remaining there long past the time that we bother to think about them, has stayed with Pete all of his life, and, in some not-fully-understood way, kept him well-stocked in negative feelings about exercise for all of his adult life.

Not anymore.

As he recounted what I've just told you, he had tears in his eyes. "That 8.5 mile for me meant more to me than you could possibly know", he said.

That got me thinking.

Pete had an inner critic telling him that he looked silly when he exercised. That he'd never be any good at it, that he "ran like a girl". What Bill Humphries had done was not just teach him how to run, but somehow get him past something that had been holding him back and keeping him imprisoned in a body which he was finally ready to leave behind.

How many of us have similar incidents, similar self-evaluations, gathering cobwebs in our minds' closets, preventing us from really breaking through and having the bodies that we want to have? Or for that matter, the relationships? Or the income? Or feeling good about the stuff we *do* have?

How many were called "Fat" and believed it was a statement about us for all time? How many believed- and still believe- that the number on the scale makes a major statement about who we are? How many are caught up in intricate entanglements of relationships that would be severely threatened if we were ever to break out of the role our weight assigns to us and become something different?

How many have people in our lives who would really be threatened if we began to shine?

Now this isn't to say that there aren't real influences on weight that all of us struggle with: genetics, hormones, dieting history, metabolism, physiology, cravings, neurotransmitter levels, you name it. But it's also worth checking out whether some of these stories we tell ourselves- the chatter of our inner voices- keep us imprisoned in the past, or in an image of ourselves that no longer serves or nurtures us.

Here are some of my candidates for the top ten list of stories from the "inner voices" that just might be holding you back regarding weight:

1. I'll always be fat

2. I'm not attractive

3. No one will ever want me at this weight

4. I have no self-control

5. It's my family's *(husband's, son's, father's, mother's, lover's, boyfriend's, girlfriend's) fault

6. I can't really be happy till I lose X pounds

7. I'm not athletic

8. I "deserve" it, it's not gonna "kill" me

9. Fat people aren't sexy

10. I'll start tomorrow

Any of them sound familiar?

If so, maybe you and that "chatterbox" in your head ought to sit down and have a heart-to-heart.

Maybe it's time for him to move out.

After   all,   he's   lived   there   long   enough.

EAT YOUR WAY TO WELLNESS
IN SIX EASY STEPS

Healthy eating is one of the cornerstones of any wellness program

For years, those of us who have been concerned with the creeping epidemic of obesity have been told that the answer is to simply "eat fewer calories". Kind of the culinary equivalent of "just saying no".

Problem is, this strategy doesn't work very well.

Many of us overeat because we are eating the wrong foods. Our bodies are over fat but undernourished. We suffer with cravings, mood swings and energy fluctuations. This in turn creates more stress in our lives, which takes us further and further from the path of wellness and balance.

There is a better solution to the problem than just cutting calories. It's a solution that's based on one of the central tenants in my Diet Boot Camp program to transform your body, your health and your life". Simply stated it goes like this: *Give the body what it needs and virtually every condition will improve.* This includes- but is not limited to- the condition of being overweight. The body has a remarkable, almost mystical ability to heal itself, *if* you give it the raw materials it needs to nourish itself: Real foods, pure water, sensible sunshine, restful sleep and rich human connections.

Simple, really.

Follow these six steps to eating your way to wellness and you may find that cravings, overeating and mood swings become a thing of the past. Your health will improve, your weight will settle to a place at which you can be comfortable and fit, and balance will be restored.

You will indeed be eating your way to wellness.

1. **Don't skip meals**. Every time you skip meals your body interprets this as an emergency of sorts, and it releases increased amounts of stress hormones. These stress hormones are your body's way of passing along the information to all the systems that there's trouble ahead. Your primitive digestion system interprets this to mean that you should store fat for the emergency your body thinks is coming. Important brain chemicals needed to feel good are depleted. You are set up for imbalance

2. **Eat a protein at every meal**. A protein serving is about the size of a deck of cards. Choose from fish, lean meats, turkey, chicken and eggs. Organic foods are likely to have less levels of toxins, hormones, antibiotics, chemicals and pesticides; organic eggs from free-range chickens have more of the heart healthy omega-3 fats.

3. **At every meal, eat a little bit of healthy fat**. This can include nuts, extra-virgin olive oil, avocado, or even a little fresh creamy butter. The difference between "good" and "bad" fats is not the difference between "saturated" and "unsaturated", it's the difference between "damaged" and "undamaged". Naturally occurring fats from real foods, which haven't been subjected to high heat, chemical processing, refining and hydrogenation are rarely the problem.

4. **At every meal add some fibrous vegetables**.

This includes broccoli, cauliflower, spinach, kale, celery, carrots, mushrooms, onions, asparagus and peppers but there are dozens of others. If you're an egg eater, try a vegetable omelet for breakfast, or some freshly made vegetable juice. Although tomatoes are technically a fruit, you can use them as part of your vegetable allowance since they fit nicely into most breakfast menus.

5. **Add a "real" carbohydrate***. These include sweet potatoes, oatmeal, beans, legumes and real, honest whole-grain breads. *(Note: This step needs to be applied really conscientiously and is actually not applicable to everyone at every meal. Some folks will do better with a grain-free diet, and others need to really limit even the "good" starchy carbs like sweet potatoes. Almost everyone can have a small portion of oatmeal for breakfast though, even diabetics)

6. **Eat some berries every day**. Raspberries, blueberries, strawberries- all are loaded with fiber, have low sugar, and are a virtual cornucopia of healthy stuff like antioxidants and phytochemicals.

When you plan your eating according to these guidelines, you will find that calorie counting is not as important, since your appetite will begin to self-regulate. You will be choosing from foods that nourish the body and soul and sustain and replenish the systems in your body that lead to good health. Weight will settle to a comfortable place and energy will increase. As you begin to eliminate foods that are over processed and refined and replace them with the real foods your body needs, your sense of balance and harmony with the things around you will be restored.

These foods may take a bit longer to prepare, but the

benefits to your health and wellness are incalculable.

Real foods, *pure* water. Take with a daily dose of sunshine, exercise and loving relationships.

It's a virtual prescription for health and well-being.

10 SUPERFOODS YOU NEED TO KNOW ABOUT

1. Blueberries

These amazing berries are on anyone's list of superfoods. Recent research shows that their brain food--feeding blueberries to rats actually slows their age-related mental decline. Blueberries contain *pterostilbene*, a plant compound recently shown to have cholesterol-lowering properties. Their ORAC value (antioxidant rating) is the highest of any fruit. And blueberries are rich in fiber. Tip: try them frozen. They taste like sherbet!

2. Guava

Among the superfoods of the world, guava is a sleeper. With a taste that's been described as "part strawberry part pear", one low-calorie cup of this vitamin rich fruit contains a whopping 8 grams of fiber. And in one widely used test of antioxidant power, guava scored second only to blueberries, and right behind kale. Guava also contains cancer fighting lycopene.

3. Kale

Kale is a member of the brassica family, vegetable royalty that boasts cabbage and broccoli among it's relatives. It's rich in potent cancer fighting substances called indoles, and loaded with bone-building vitamin K. Kale also contains *sulforaphane*, a powerful nutrient that helps the liver detoxify carcinogens and other toxins. Kale has the highest antioxidant rating of any vegetable and is ridiculously low in calories. Try it tossed with olive oil, a few dried cranberries and some pine nuts.

4. Sardines

The best kept secret in the world when it comes to health foods and the secret weapon of travelers looking for a cheap, portable, easily available source of protein. Sardines are rich in omega-3 fats, and one of the least contaminated of any seafood since it's so low on the food chain. Eat them out of the can or throw them on some salad.

5. Apples

Apples come under the heading of "things your grandmother was right about". The apple's reputation for keeping you out of the doctor's office is well deserved. It's loaded with pectin (an important fiber), and one of the best sources of boron, a little known nutrient that helps support strong and healthy bones. An apple with a glass of water is a great natural appetite suppressant. Highest antioxidant value: red delicious.

6. Coconut oil

This superb oil has been long neglected as a healthy oil because it contains saturated fat. But not to worry: the saturated fat in coconut is a very healthy kind called MCT (medium chain triglycerides) which is easily burned by the body for energy. Coconut oil also contains lauric acid, a natural anti-viral and anti-microbial. And today's excellent virgin coconut oil- unlike the inferior products of a few decades ago- doesn't contain trans fats. Note to skeptics: The Puka Puka islanders consumed 80 % of their diet from coconut products and had virtually no heart disease.

7. Green tea

Here's a superstar beverage if there ever was one. Green tea helps with weight loss and helps fight against cancer. It contains EGCG, a catechin (plant compound) which stimulates metabolism and has anti-cancer properties to boot. Green tea also contains theanine, a natural relaxant which helps explain why the caffeine in green tea doesn't make you nearly as jittery as coffee.

8. Flaxseeds

Flaxseed oil is one of the only plant sources of omega-3 fats, but the flaxseeds themselves provide the added benefit of fiber along with the omega-3's. Flaxseeds can be thrown on salads, tossed into smoothies, or sprinkled on vegetables. They also contain lignans, a group of plant nutrients that have been studied by the National Cancer Institute for their cancer preventive properties.

9. Eggs

The protein source against which all others are judged. And for goodness sake, stop with the egg white omlettes. The yolk is loaded with good stuff! Half of the measly 4.5 grams of fat are actually monounsaturated fat, the same heart-healthy fat that's in olive oil. The yolks are also one of the best sources of *lutein*, the superstar of eye nutrition. Plus they contain *choline*, which helps support brain function and help keep harmful homocysteine levels down.

Look for the new designer eggs with increased omega-3 content.

10. Pomegranate juice

If you're wondering if all the hype about pomegranate juice is for real, stop wondering: it is. Animal studies suggest that pomegranate juice combats artherogenesis (hardening of the arteries) as well as other cardiovascular diseases such as strokes and heart attacks. It's rich in antioxidants and has a higher amount of *polyphenols*- heart healthy plant compounds-- than even red wine. Look for the pure pomegranate juice (not the watered down cocktail). You can always dilute it with water or mix it with other juices.

IT'S ALL ABOUT THE CALORIES, RIGHT?

Gather round, folks, cause I'm gonna tell you a story.

Once upon a time- around 1890 actually- a scientist named Wilbur Atwater got the bright idea of putting food into a special machine, burning it and measuring the amount of heat it produced. The machine was called a calorimeter, and old Wilbur decided to call the energy produced by burning the food into ash "calories". Thus he was able to figure how many calories were contained in just about any food you could think of.

Shortly afterwards, scientists applied the same concept to exercise. Using a few calculations, they soon figured out how many calories were "burned" doing everything from sleeping to cross-country skiing.

Within no time, an idea was born: weight gain happened when a person *took in* more calories than he *burned up*. The body, it was reasoned, behaves like a calorimeter. Put in calories (from food) use up calories (from living, exercising, digesting, etc) and look at your balance sheet. If more is coming in than going out, you gain weight. If more goes out than came in, you lose. Simple. Especially if the body behaved like a calorimeter.

But it doesn't.

The people who sell empty, useless, nutritionally dead calories- sugar anyone?- love the calorie theory. According to them, since weight loss is only a matter of eating less calories, sugar is perfectly acceptable. Just don't eat so many darn calories and you won't get fat. If you do, says the sugar industry, don't blame us. Sugar doesn't cause weight gain, as long as you don't eat more calories than you "burn".

'Course that ignores all the other things that sugar does besides provide (empty) calories: like raise blood sugar, depress the immune system, rob the body of calcium and use up mineral stores. But that's another story.

Then there's one other itty bitty problem: the body *doesn't* behave like a calorimeter. It behaves like a chemistry lab.

Here's an example: Eat a bar that's 100 calories of sugar. Your blood sugar jumps up. The pancreas responds with a big shot of insulin, whose job it is to bring blood sugar down. In some people it doesn't do such a great job, leaving them with high blood sugar and high insulin, both risk factors for heart disease. In others it does the job OK, but the sugar winds up in the fat cells. Either way, you lose. And we're not talking about losing fat!

On the other hand, let's say you eat a bar that's 100

calories of protein, fat and fiber. The protein provides nutrients necessary for the building of the body's architecture- bones, muscles, enzymes, neurotransmitters. It also makes you feel full so you're less likely to overeat. The fiber slows the entrance of sugar into the bloodstream. The fat provides important building blocks for cell membranes and hormones. Protein has only a mild effect on blood sugar and insulin, and neither fiber nor fat have any effect at all. While both bars are equal from a *calorie* point of view, they are anything *but* equal from the point of view of hormones, fat storage and health.

The effect of different sources of calories on blood sugar and hormones like insulin is one of the most important concepts in nutrition, and one which dietitians still haven't figured out

The bottom line: Eat foods that have the least impact on blood sugar- fiber, for example, and fat, along with green leafy vegetables, low sugar fruit and plenty of protein, all of which provide nutrients, building blocks and health benefits. Sugar on the other hand provides none of those, and will instead keep you on the blood sugar roller coaster that inevitably leads to health problems such as obesity.

So if you're looking only at calories, you're missing the fine print. Take two typical "low carb bars. While both have about 200 calories, Bar One has only 1 measly gram of fiber, 14 grams of protein, and 20 grams of sugar alcohols. Bar Two, on the other hand, has a whopping 10 grams of fiber, 19 grams of protein and a mere 4 grams of sugar alcohols, a sweetener which *usually* does not have a significant impact on blood sugar or insulin.

That's the fine print that's missing if you only pay attention to calories. Calories *do* matter- but they're very far from the whole story.

Remember, God is in the details- or in this case, in the fine print.

WHY STRESS MATTERS

Suppose I told you that there was one action you could take right now that could improve your chances of losing weight permanently, and that taking that particular action wouldn't be painful, expensive or difficult.

Now that I've got your attention….

Suppose I *also* told you that you wouldn't need any special equipment to do it, you wouldn't have to take any special pills or metabolic enhancers, and that you could do this particular activity right in your own home. In fact, right in your own *bed*.

Not only *that*, you wouldn't have to learn any special new skills- you already know how to do this particular activity as well as anyone else on the planet.

Interested? I thought so.

Well, there *is* such an activity, and it's called…...

Sleep.

Yup. Plain old fashioned, garden-variety nighttime shut-eye. Deep, undisturbed, warm, fuzzy, refreshing sleep. The kind most of us don't get nearly enough of. And, strange as it may seem, not getting enough can be sabotaging your weight loss efforts, not to mention your overall health.

Big time.

Here's why: On top of the kidneys are two little walnut sized glands called the "adrenals". These glands secrete important hormones - one of the most important of these being cortisol. Cortisol is also known as a "stress hormone". It's secreted in times of emergency, along with a related hormone we all know about called adrenaline. Although cortisol is needed by every cell in the body, problems arise when we secrete too much of it. Our active, complicated, over-committed, time-crunched lives cause us to produce a virtual flood of it; only know are we beginning to fully understand the consequences and health implications of this situation.

Excess cortisol is in effect an "emergency warning system" that tells the body something's coming that's going to require a lot of energy. Stress hormones are the body's way of preparing you for action, such as running from or fighting off a predator. That's why stress hormones are known as the "fight or flight" hormones. Among its other missions, cortisol signals the body to store fat. It tells the body to break down protein (muscle) for energy, but hold on to fat for dear life. Consistently elevated levels of cortisol can lower your metabolic rate and can also lead to brain aging and cognitive impairment. (Now you know why you don't think so clearly when you're overtired and overstressed!)

While most people are aware of dozens of "stressors" in

their life- jobs, families, relationships, bosses, traffic and all the other usual suspects- many people do *not* know that one of the biggest stressors of all is not getting enough sleep.

Followed closely by dieting.

Ironic, isn't it? Dieting, especially of the very low-calorie, low-protein kind, *raises* the very hormone responsible for fighting fat loss!

When you don't sleep enough to feel fully and completely rested and refreshed- and who among us does?- you also interfere with the nightly secretion of another hormone- HGH (Human Growth Hormone), which is secreted during the deepest levels of REM (rapid eye movement) sleep. HGH signals the body to hold on to valuable muscle and to burn fat.

Beginning to get the picture?

When people ask me to characterize my Diet Boot Camp program in a few words, the phrase I usually use is "holistic weight loss". Here's why: The biggest problem with conventional weight loss programs is that they treat the topic of losing weight as if it's a math problem- all you have to do is count the calories (or fat grams, or carbohydrate grams) and bingo, you're home free. Sorry, Cholly.

It's not that simple.

Your weight is intimately related to everything else in your life. Your stress levels are a big player in this game, and they in turn are influenced not only by how much you sleep, but by your relationships, your connectedness to your community, your friends, your family, your spiritual center, even your pets.

So the next time a stressed out friend asks you for a suggestion about the best way to lose weight fast, maybe you ought to say….

"Hey. Take a nice warm bath, put on some Mozart and a nice peaceful nap. Have a nice cool glass of water. Relax. Treat yourself like a queen for a while and take a breather from worrying".

You wouldn't be far wrong.

FALLING OFF THE DIET WAGON

One of the most discouraging aspects of weight loss is the inevitable slips. Everyone has them. For some people, an occasional "slip" engenders an all-out binge, followed by guilt, self-recrimination, and a sense of powerlessness and a feeling of "what's the use?"

Sound familiar?

I call it "falling off the diet wagon", and if you change how you think about it, you don't need to be victimized by it anymore.

To illustrate what I'm talking about, let's look at a simple children's board game called "Chutes and Ladders". Here's how it works: you use a spinner to advance over 100 spaces on the board. Every so often, there are ladders, which leapfrog you over a lot of spaces, advancing you towards the winners spot. However, equally prominent along the path are chutes, which send the player back in the opposite direction.

Some kids play this game with a laissez faire, "whatever"

attitude, taking life as it comes with all its ups and downs, pitfalls and triumphs. They learn the wonderful moral of the game, which is that half of the secret to life is just showing up: keep playing the game, and eventually you'll get where you're going.

Some, however, get very upset when they land on a chute. They're ready to quit the game, pick up their proverbial marbles and go home. For some reason, they "believe" that life isn't supposed to have any chutes, so when they land on them they are very disappointed and feel like giving up.

Weight loss is like a huge game of chutes and ladders.

In dealing with hundreds of clients over the years, I've discovered that the biggest difference between the winners and the losers in the weight loss wars isn't really whether or not people have "slips" and go off their program. (In fact, it's not really a question of "if" they have them, it's a question of "when", since just about everyone has them).

What really makes the difference is how you deal with them when they happen.

Here's an example: You've been absolutely wonderful on your eating plan for three weeks, sticking to your exercise routine and feeling pretty terrific. You go to your best friend's wedding, and have a glass of wine. Before you know it, someone is insisting you try those delicious little canapes, and before the wedding singer can say "Tanta Elka Cuts the Cake", you've managed to down about 4000 unwanted calories from stuff you wouldn't have been caught dead looking at during the past couple of weeks:

pates, deserts, breads, you name it.

Most people think that's where the action stops. Actually, it's where the real action begins.

First, a reality check. Have you done a lot of damage? Not really. Maybe you put on a pound or two. Big deal. You can knock it off in no time, and go right back to "work" on yourself.

So what's the problem?

The problem isn't what we did, but what we make it "mean". We tell ourselves that our "transgression" means that we have no will power, that we will never succeed, that our efforts are in vain.

In other words, we hit a chute and now we want to stop the game.

Let me suggest something more empowering.

Suppose, instead, we learn to see life's occasional "chutes" as just that, stumbling blocks that everyone hits on their personal path to personal power, nothing to be afraid of, and certainly nothing to give a lot of "meaning" to.

So you hit a chute. Next roll of the dice, you might hit a ladder.

Most important of all, you can't win the game unless you keep on playing. And every minute gives you a new chance for another flick of the spinner.

Take it. And don't look back.

ABOUT THE AUTHOR

Jonny Bowden, PhD, CNS, (aka "The Rogue Nutritionist") is a nationally known expert on weight loss, nutrition and health. He is a board-certified nutritionist with a master's degree in psychology and the author of thirteen books on health, healing, food and longevity including two best-sellers, "The 150 Healthiest Foods on Earth" and "Living Low Carb". A frequent guest on television and radio, he has appeared on Fox News, CNN, MSNBC, ABC, NBC, and CBS as an expert on nutrition, weight loss, and longevity. He is a past member of the Editorial Advisory Board for Men's Health magazine, is the Nutrition Editor for Pilates Style, and is a regular contributor to AOL, *Vanity Fair Online, Clean Eating Magazine, Better Nutrition,* and *Total Health Magazine Online.*

Dr. Jonny has contributed to articles for dozens of national publications (print and online) including *The New York Times, The Wall Street Journal, Forbes, The Daily Beast, The Huffington Post, Vanity Fair Online, Time, Oxygen, Marie Claire, Diabetes Focus, GQ, US Weekly, Cosmopolitan, Self, Fitness, Family Circle, Allure, Men's Heath, Prevention, In Style, Natural Health,* and many other publications. He appears regularly as an expert on ABC-TV Los Angeles.

He is the author of:

- "The 150 Healthiest Foods on Earth"
- "The 100 Healthiest Foods for Pregnancy" (with Allison Tannis)
- "The Most Effective Natural Cures on Earth"
- "The Healthiest Meals on Earth" (with Jeannette Bessinger)
- "The 150 Most Effective Ways to Boost Your Energy"
- "The Most Effective Ways to Live Longer"
- "The Live Longer Cookbook" (with Jeannette Bessinger)
- "Living Low Carb" (Revised and expanded edition) (100,000 in print and winner of the "Consumer Nutrition Book of the Year" award)
- "The Healthiest 15-Minute Recipes on Earth" (with Jeannette Bessinger)

Dr. Bowden has a Master's Degree in psychology and counseling and a PhD in nutrition, and has earned six national certifications in personal training and exercise. He is board certified by the American College of Nutrition, a member of the American Society for Nutrition, and a much in-demand speaker at conferences and events across the country.

CHECK OUT MY LATEST BOOK!

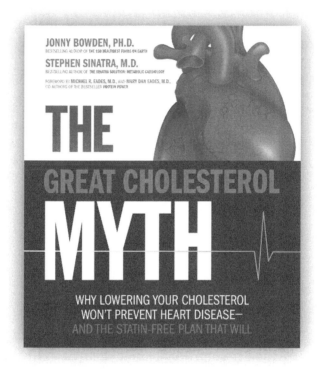

Heart disease is the #1 killer.

However, traditional heart disease protocols--with their emphasis on lowering cholesterol--have it all wrong.

Emerging science is showing that cholesterol levels are a poor predictor of heart disease and that standard prescriptions for lowering it, such as ineffective low-fat/high-carb diets and serious, side-effect-causing statin drugs, obscure the real causes of heart disease.

Even doctors at leading institutions have been misled

for years based on creative reporting of research results from pharmaceutical companies intent on supporting the $31-billion-a-year cholesterol-lowering drug industry.

RAVE REVIEWS

"The Great Cholesterol Myth finally sheds light on the true story, why millions are being harmed by statin drugs and how to really prevent heart disease. Everyone with heart disease, on a statin, or with a family history of heart disease must read this book. And if your doctor recommends a statin, read this book first!"

—Mark Hyman, M.D., best-selling author of The Blood Sugar Solution

" If you want to know the truth about cholesterol, and what you absolutely must do to improve your heart health, this is the book for you. Jonny Bowden and Dr. Stephen Sinatra reveal the facts in a compelling and insightful way. This invaluable book belongs on the bookshelf of anyone who cares about the truth in medicine and healing."

—Daniel Amen, M.D., CEO, Amen Clinics, Inc., author of Use Your Brain to Change Your Age

" The book you're holding is dangerous, and may even upset you. That's because everything you know about cholesterol is probably wrong. Doctors Jonny Bowden and Stephen Sinatra provide both the science to vindicate this unfairly demonized molecule and a plan of action so you can attain optimal health."

—JJ Virgin, best-selling author of The Virgin Diet

Get your copy at Amazon.com

Made in the USA
San Bernardino, CA
03 February 2014